5 minute first aid for children

British Red Cross

Caring for people in crisis

5 minute first aid

for children

Hodder Arnold

A MEMBER OF THE HODDER HEADLINE GROUP

Orders: Please contact Bookpoint Ltd, 130 Milton Park, Abingdon, Oxon OX14 4SB. Telephone: (44) 01235 827720, Fax: (44) 01235 400454. Lines are open from 9.00 to 18.00, Monday to Saturday, with a 24-hour message answering service. You can also order through our website www.hoddereducation.com

British Library Cataloguing in Publication Data
A catalogue record for this title is available from the British Library.

ISBN-10: 0 340 90461 5
ISBN-13: 9 780340 904619

First published	2005
Impression number	10 9 8 7 6 5 4 3 2 1
Year	2008 2007 2006 2005

Typeset by Transet Limited, Coventry, England.
Printed in Great Britain for Hodder Arnold, a division of Hodder Headline, 338 Euston Road, London NW1 3BH, by Cox & Wyman Ltd, Reading, Berkshire.

Hodder Headline's policy is to use papers that are natural, renewable and recyclable products and made from wood grown in sustainable forests. The logging and manufacturing processes are expected to conform to the environmental regulations of the country of origin.

contents

acknowledgements

The authors would like to pay special thanks to Charlotte Hall, Catherine Jones, Genevieve Okech and Naomi Safir.

preface

The British Red Cross, as part of the International Red Cross and Red Crescent Movement, is the world's largest first-aid training organization. With over 180 Red Cross societies worldwide we endeavour to make first-aid knowledge and skills accessible to individuals, families, schools and the wider community.

You never know when someone may need your help but it is highly likely that when called on to provide emergency first aid it will be to someone close to you such as a friend or a member of your own family. Therefore, we have produced the *Five-minute First Aid* series in order to give you the relevant skills and confidence needed to be able to save a life and help an injured person, whatever your situation.

We appreciate that it is difficult to find time in hectic lifestyles to learn first-aid skills. Consequently, this series is designed so that you can learn and absorb each specific, essential skill that is relevant to you in just five minutes, and you can pick up and put down the book as you wish. The features throughout the book will help you to reinforce what you have learnt and will build your confidence in applying first aid.

This book is divided into five-minute sections, so that you can discover each invaluable skill in just a short amount of time.

one-minute wonder

One-minute wonders ask and answer the questions that you might be thinking as you read.

key skills

The key-skills features emphasize and reiterate the main skills of the section – helping you to commit them to memory and recall them when called upon to do so.

summary

Summary sections summarize the key points of the chapter in order to further consolidate your knowledge and understanding.

self-testers

The self-testers ensure that you have learnt the most important facts of the chapter. They will give you an indication of how much you are absorbing as you go along and help to build your confidence. (Note: some of the multiple choice questions may have more than one possible answer!)

We hope that this book will give you the opportunity to learn the most important skills you will ever need in a friendly, straightforward way, and that it prepares you for any first-aid situation that you may encounter.

introduction

We all recognize that accidents and injuries are a part of growing up. A few weeks after we are born, we start learning and exploring. While parents and carers take many precautions to stop accidents happening, accidents are an inevitable part of a child's development. We all know that 'prevention is better than cure', but it is impossible to monitor your children all the time and, while some accidents are preventable, it is important to remember that a child's enquiring mind will, on occasions, result in him hurting or injuring himself. Thankfully, most injuries received by children are minor ones that can be treated at home or by specialist advice from health professionals. However, there are some illnesses and injuries that require prompt and appropriate action from the first person on the scene and that may be you, the child's parent or carer.

In recent years, we have become more aware of the importance of 'immediate care' or first aid, and we now understand the importance of that initial response. In some cases, the care a child receives in the first minutes after an accident can be the difference between life and death. In other cases, immediate care can prevent the condition getting worse, reduce the pain and speed up the child's recovery.

We in the British Red Cross have been delivering first aid and teaching it for over 100 years. Our research tells us that parents and carers of young children are more likely to be called upon to deliver first aid and despite the well-known phrase that 'a little knowledge is a dangerous thing', we know that a little first-aid knowledge can make a big difference to your child. Our aim is not to try and turn you into a medical professional. As you will appreciate, doctors and nurses concentrate on diagnosis and long-term treatment. All that is required of you after reading this book is to make some very basic observations of your child in the event of him requiring first aid; we do not expect you to make a detailed clinical diagnosis, and that is why we have concentrated on initial treatment rather than diagnosis. As an example of this, in Chapter 7 we describe the treatment of a sprain and a strain but, we only make a passing reference to the difference between the two because the initial treatment is the same. Remember that first aid, as the name suggests, is the first care a child receives, it's about you doing your best using the knowledge and skills gained from this book.

The chances of making a situation worse are slim if you act in accordance with the guidance given in the book. Keeping calm and acting in a logical manner is key to providing the right treatment.

We recognize that there is a lot to remember; all we hope is that you recall the key part of the treatment described. For example, if a child is not breathing, you can breathe for him. If he is losing a lot of blood, try and stop it. If he has a burn, cool it. Much of this is common sense and we have added extra advice to make the treatment more effective.

When asking parents 'What would you do when faced with an emergency?', their response tends to be 'I'd panic' or 'I'd call an ambulance'. These responses are understandable but, as you will be aware after reading this book, there are some important things that can be done before the ambulance arrives, or while waiting for medical advice.

A sense of panic on discovering that your child is unwell is not uncommon, but using your common sense and acting in a logical manner is key to dealing with any emergency situation.

The guidance in this book relates to the treatment of children (1–7 years old inclusive). We would like to point out that in the areas of resuscitation and choking different procedures apply to babies (0–1 year old) and children over 7 years old. These procedures are referred to in detail in *Five-Minute First Aid for Babies* and *Five-Minute First Aid Life-Saving Skills*.

For convenience and clarity, we use the pronoun 'he' throughout the book when referring to the injured child.

1

how to deal with an emergency

If a job description existed for being a parent it would contain a long list of things you may be required to do in the role. Many of these would be predictable, like feeding the child, keeping him warm, giving him love and caring for him when he is unwell. Others would not be as predictable and these include being prepared to respond in an emergency situation. Many of us, whether parents or carers, would prefer not to have to think about an emergency situation involving our children. However, the reality is that accidents happen, and injuries and illness may result from these.

It is virtually impossible to predict how any of us will respond in any given emergency, especially one involving our children. We all recognize that prevention is better than cure, yet however safety-conscious we are, it is impossible to completely rule out the chances of an accident happening, whether at home or in the garden, on the road or on the beach. It is important that we do not end up as paranoid parents. Acknowledge that climbing trees in the park or diving into the local lagoon may present a risk to your child, but realize that they are also an important part of his development. The last thing we want to do is wrap our children up in cotton wool and deprive them of taking some of the risks that make growing up fun. We also appreciate that most accidents are minor ones and simply require a bit of common sense, possibly a plaster and a cuddle. Others are much more critical, and the actions of the first person on the scene can make a huge difference.

In this book we have tried to take a practical view of having to respond to an emergency. We have highlighted the things you should do, some of the things you should not do, and give advice that is based on our clinical knowledge and our experience as parents. We realize that it may not be possible for you to retain all the guidance contained in the book, and therefore we have highlighted the key skills and answered the kind of questions we are asked when teaching first aid.

It is difficult to provide definitive guidance on how to respond in every situation involving your child because the situations may range from a minor burn to discovering your child cannot be seen in your newly landscaped garden with water feature. Therefore, we have focused on some of the things you should consider and do, whatever the emergency.

an emergency situation

In an emergency situation, approach the child and assess the situation. Try to work out what has happened and how, and think of your own safety. Often the cause of the accident will be obvious to you. If you have been ironing and leave the room and you suddenly hear your child scream, on returning to the room you find the ironing board on its side, your child, obviously distressed, sitting on the floor while the iron burns a nice iron-shaped mark into your carpet. You don't have to be an amateur detective to work this one out. Or do you? Has your child suffered a head injury as a result of the ironing board falling on him; has he touched the iron and been burnt; or has the tangled and frayed flex you meant to replace resulted in an electrical injury to your child. Whatever the cause and the resulting injuries, you should first ask the following questions:

- Is there any danger?
- Is there anybody around who can help?

Don't be reluctant to call the neighbours or passers-by. Ask yourself whether this situation requires an ambulance. First aid is all about using the resources that are available to you, and that includes bystanders. If in doubt call 999 (or 112 in Europe) for an ambulance, or get someone else to do it. Other situations may be much more complex and potentially serious than this, but the same principles apply.

Remember when calling for an ambulance to give the location of the incident, the age of the child and any information about the condition or overall well-being of the child. This is helpful to the ambulance service in terms of prioritizing the call. The ambulance controller may ask you questions like:

- Is the child conscious?
- Is he breathing?
- Does he look distressed?
- What colour is his skin?

It is therefore important to pass on any information you think may be helpful. While you are waiting for the ambulance to arrive, continue to monitor the child's condition, observe his colouring, his breathing, the temperature of his skin. Equally important is the need to reassure the child; keep talking in a calm and reassuring manner, touch him on the head or face or cradle him if possible. People who have found themselves in this situation say the time seems to go very slowly if you are waiting for an ambulance – this is probably because you want your child to have the best care possible as quickly as possible. Ambulance personnel often insist that a parent or carer travels with the child in the ambulance to the hospital. They may, however, be unable to carry siblings and so if you have other children, you should try and make baby-sitting arrangements for while you are away. In most cases your consent for the treatment will be needed once your child is in the accident and emergency department.

While a child's condition can improve quickly, it can also deteriorate in a short period of time. Even if the child's condition improves while you are waiting for the ambulance, it is probably best to allow the ambulance to attend and to obtain a professional opinion. In some situations the child's condition may improve and then deteriorate. Ambulance paramedics are understanding people and remember that many of them are parents like you.

You may find that talking to the child and continuing to reassure him is not only helpful to the child, it also helps to keep you calm. Once the emergency is over, it is important to talk about it with friends, family and other parents to share your experience and feelings.

***one-minute** wonder*

Q Is it true that I can be sued if the first aid I give does not work?

A No. As long as you are using treatment that is likely to be of most benefit to the injured child, the principle of the 'Good Samaritan' supports those who deliver first aid within accepted boundaries. In the majority of cases of first aid being delivered to children, the child will be known to you.

Some people are concerned about getting an infection when performing first aid, especially if there is blood involved or if they have to do rescue breathing. The risk of getting an infection in this way is small. Some procedures can help reduce the risk of infection, for example,washing your hands after treatment, using gloves if they are available, covering cuts with waterproof plasters and having access to appropriate equipment. See the recommended contents of a first-aid kit on page 119.

key skills

When faced with an emergency situation, remember to:

- keep calm
- assess the situation
- ensure your safety
- continue to monitor the baby's condition
- ask others to help you.

If in doubt, call for an ambulance. Remember, never put yourself in danger.

one-minute wonder

Q You mention the importance of calling 999 (or 112 in Europe) for an ambulance. How will I know when to call an ambulance?

A This depends on the type of emergency and the condition of the child. Trust your instincts as a parent and, if in doubt, make that call.

one-minute wonder

Q Will I be charged if I call an ambulance unnecessarily?

A No. It is unlikely that you will be charged for calling an emergency ambulance. However, the charging policy varies depending on the ambulance trust. If an ambulance is necessary, please do not make the cost of an ambulance a reason not to make the call.

5 5

The following advice should help you in ensuring a logical response to any accident involving a child. This SAMPLE pneumonic may help you to remember some of the key points to consider when carrying out the initial assessment of a child in a first-aid situation.

S – Signs and symptoms. In the context of first aid, we use the term 'signs and symptoms'. Signs are what you or the carer, as the first aider, observes. The symptoms are what the child feels and how he tells you he feels.

A – Allergies. Is the child allergic to anything? Remember, many young children now carry alert bracelets advising first aiders and medical staff in the event of an accident of what they are allergic to. This can include medications like penicillin. It can also include information with regards to their condition. For example, does the child have epilepsy, diabetes or other conditions that need to be considered as part of the treatment?

M – Medication. Is the child on any medication? If so, what is it and when did he last take it? In the context of first aid, we do not expect you to have comprehensive knowledge and understanding of medication, but this information is important when you are reporting to ambulance crew or health-care professionals.

P – Child's past history. In some first-aid situations, it is important to know if the child has any relevant medical history that may inform his treatment. For example, has the child collapsed previously and, if so, why?

L – Last oral intake. When did the child last eat or drink? This information is important to the hospital staff when considering further treatment.

E – Events. Always consider the events leading up to an injury or an illness. What happened before you arrived on the scene?

priorities of treatment

After having ensured your own safety, the priority in any first-aid situation is to make sure that the child can breathe. To maintain life we need to be able to breathe, and to be able to breathe we must make sure the passage from the back of the throat to the lungs, known as the airway, is open. There is a large number of things that can block the airway therefore affecting a child's ability to breathe.

These include:

- choking
- the child falling unconscious for whatever reason and the tongue falling to the back of the throat and blocking the airway
- tipping the head back when treating a nose bleed; the blood can run down the back of the throat and result in the child having difficulty in breathing.

The open airway and breathing ensure that the body gets enough oxygen, but the oxygen needs to be circulated around the body in the blood stream. This is known as the circulation. We make many references to the ABC throughout this book:

A for airway
B for breathing
C for circulation, to ensure that blood gets around the body to keep the key organs alive.

In addition to these priorities, you should check to see if there is any evidence of serious bleeding both internal and external (see Chapter 3), and then check for any obvious injuries.

In this book we use a variety of terms to describe the need to get some assistance: 'seek help', 'get medical advice', and 'call 999 (or 112 in Europe) for an ambulance'. In terms of seeking help, this can be gained from passers-by, other members of the family or some other people who have some knowledge and expertise and may be in a position to help you.

You can ask for advice or help from specialist practitioners or first contact practitioners who may be based at your doctor's surgery, in your clinic, or via telephone or website from NHS Direct (see page 132). In the vast majority of cases involving first aid, we strongly recommend that the individual seeks medical advice or for a child, that you or anybody else seeks medical advice on their behalf. This may be from a hospital, from your local doctor or any other relevant health-care professional. For the majority of instances in which you provide care, we advise that you call for an ambulance and continue to monitor the child for a period of time after the incident, even if he has not received medical attention.

recording information

Gathering information about the child you are caring for and recording the treatment you have provided is very important. The ability to report is now seen as a key part of the role of the first aider. The information you will require from the child, if possible, is a name and address. Make some notes about the history of the accident, the injuries that you suspect, and the treatment you have given. Also record anything you have observed with regards to the child's condition when you have been treating him and, in particular, any unusual behaviour he may have exhibited throughout the treatment. We recognize that the first aider's priority is to provide the care. However, this kind of information can often be beneficial as part of the ongoing treatment in hospital or by a doctor.

road traffic accident

Road traffic accidents remain one of the most common types of accident involving young children. The priority when dealing with a road traffic accident is the same as in any other situation – ensure your own safety. It is important to protect the scene by using any visible warning signs like warning triangles or by placing vehicles in what we describe as the 'fend-off position'. Make sure that if the road is still being used and vehicles are still passing by, that they are aware of your presence and the fact that an accident has occurred. In terms of your own safety, also be aware of the presence of glass, inflammable liquids and other hazardous chemicals.

Once you have made sure that the scene is safe, check on the number and condition of the injured people. It is normal procedure for you, as a first aider, to check on the well-being of those who are quiet as they may be at a greater risk due to unconsciousness (see Chapter 2). If a child at the scene of an accident is screaming and calling for help, while his condition may be serious, at least you know that there is no risk to him associated with being unconscious.

Once you have ascertained the number and the severity of the injured people, send for help. Ask a bystander or somebody else to call for an ambulance and ensure that they pass on the relevant information about the people to the ambulance control.

While the temptation may be to get involved and start providing treatment immediately, it is important to ensure that the emergency services are on their way. Consider the needs of other services, primarily the police and the fire services. It is helpful to all the emergency authorities if the call is made at the same time. Once you have ascertained the severity of the injuries sustained by everyone, provide treatment in order of priority, starting with the most severely injured.

key skills

When dealing with any accident, and in particular a road traffic accident, ensure that the scene is safe, assess the number and potential severity of the injuries to the people involved. Dial 999 (or 112 in Europe) for the emergency services and begin treatment, dealing with the most severely injured first.

one-minute wonder

Q If I am treating a child in the middle of the road, should I move him first?

A It is important that you do not move the child until you have assessed his injuries. If you suspect a back or neck injury, you must not move him at all. Instead ask bystanders to stop the traffic.

summary

If you are the first person on the scene of any emergency situation:

- don't walk by
- get involved
- try and remain calm
- remember the key things like ABC and SAMPLE
- take charge and ask bystanders to help
- dial 999 (or 112 in Europe)
- do not take unacceptable risks.

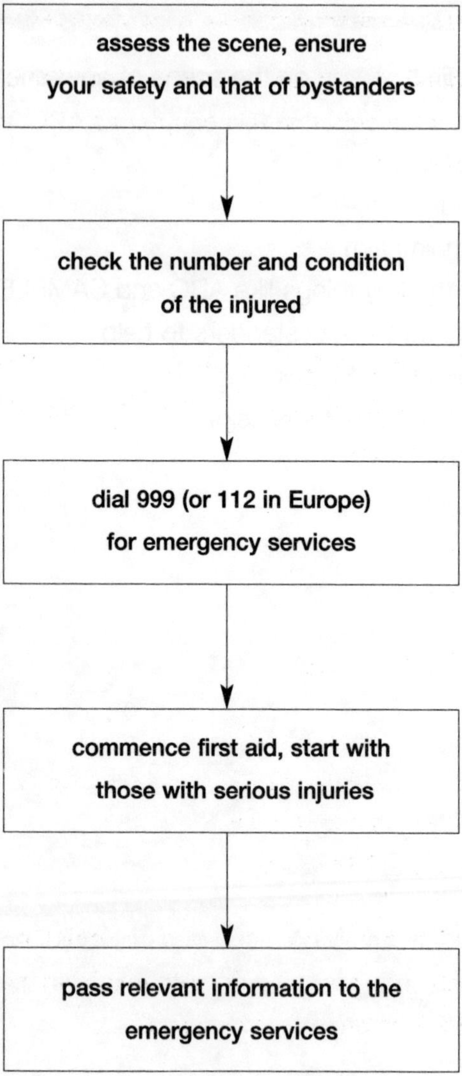

assess the scene, ensure your safety and that of bystanders
check the number and condition of the injured
dial 999 (or 112 in Europe) for emergency services
commence first aid, start with those with serious injuries
pass relevant information to the emergency services

On approaching an emergency situation

self-testers

1 In the context of first aid, when assessing the child, the priority treatment is described in this chapter as ABC. What do these letters stand for?

A ________

B ________

C ________

2 The pneumonic SAMPLE is used to describe some key considerations when assessing a child in a first-aid situation. What do the letters stand for?

S ________

A ________

M ________

P ________

L ________

E ________

3 In a first-aid situation, what is most important?

a your safety as a first aider

b the injured child's safety

4 In an accident involving more than one child, one is screaming for your attention and help, the other is lying motionless on the road. Which one should you assist first?

answers

1 **A**irway

Breathing

Circulation

2 **S**igns and symptoms

Allergies

Medication

Person's past history

Last oral intake

Events

3 **a**

4 the one lying motionless on the road

2

how to resuscitate

If your child collapses for whatever reason (which could include falls from a height, traffic accidents or as a result of a medical condition), in this chapter you will learn how to:

- check if your child is unconscious
- put him in the recovery position
- carry out rescue breathing
- give chest compressions.

conscious or unconscious?

The easiest way to check if your child is unconscious is to call out his name. If he does not respond by moving, opening his eyes or talking, try to provoke a response by tapping him on the shoulder. You should not shake a child to see if he is unconscious because there is a risk of causing further injury, such as brain injury.

If he does not respond in a coherent way, assume he is unconscious. He will appear floppy and lifeless and may have a bluish tint to his skin, particularly the lips. We often hear people use the terms 'partially conscious' or 'semi-conscious'; such descriptions are not used in the context of first aid. There are differing levels of consciousness but these are complex to assess and can alter very quickly. In terms of your role as a first aider, you just need to decide if the child is conscious or not. If in doubt regarding his response, be safe and place him in the recovery position (see page 21).

one-minute wonder

Q You refer to an unconscious child as having a bluish tint to the skin. I care for a number of children from a black or minority ethnic (BME) background. Is the bluish tint you describe as obvious in these children?

A No, you will probably notice this more in a child who has a pale complexion. If you need to check for the bluish tint, it is recommended you pull the child's lip forward and check the inside.

is the child breathing?

Once you have ascertained that the child is unconscious, you must then check if he is breathing. If you are alone, you should shout for help before checking the breathing.

To check breathing, you must first open the airway. This is the passage which air passes through from the nose and mouth into the lungs. When a child is unconscious, there is a risk that the tongue will fall to the back of his throat and block the airway, resulting in the child being unable to breathe. The airway can also become blocked by vomit, mucus or blood, especially if the child has an injury to the face.

how to open a child's airway

Assuming the child is laying on his back or side, place one hand on the child's forehead and tilt the head back. Take a quick look in the child's mouth and remove any obvious obstruction like displaced teeth from the mouth. Lift the chin using your index and middle fingers (see Figure 1).

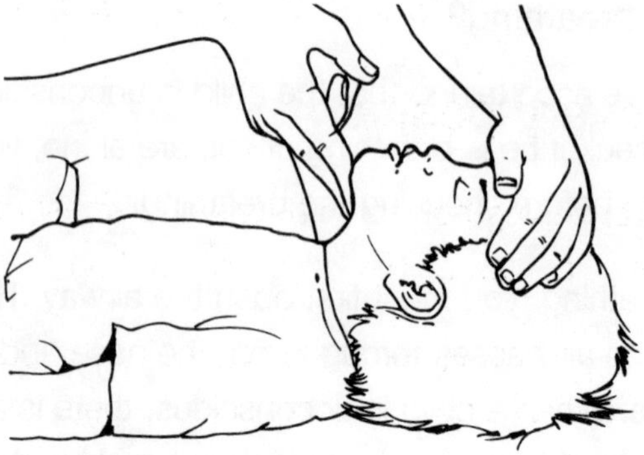

Fig 1 How to open the airway

Place your hand on the forehead and your fingertips under the chin and gently tilt the head back.

key skills

To open a child's airway, remember it is a head tilt and a chin tilt. Once the airway is open, it is now possible to check if the child is breathing. To check if a child is breathing, look, listen and feel. You do this by placing your cheek close to the child's face; you may then be able to hear breathing or feel breath on your cheek. You can also look at the child's chest to see if there is any movement. If the child is breathing, place him in the recovery position (see opposite) and call for an ambulance.

Don't rush the breathing check, allow up to ten seconds until you are sure that you know whether the child is breathing or not.

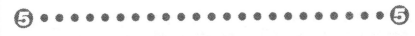

5

the recovery position

If a child is breathing but unconscious, the safest position to place him in is known as the 'recovery position'.

In the recovery position the child's airway will remain open as it allows the tongue to fall forward and also allows vomit, blood or any other fluids to drain away. If the child is already laying on his side, modify the position as shown in Figure 2.

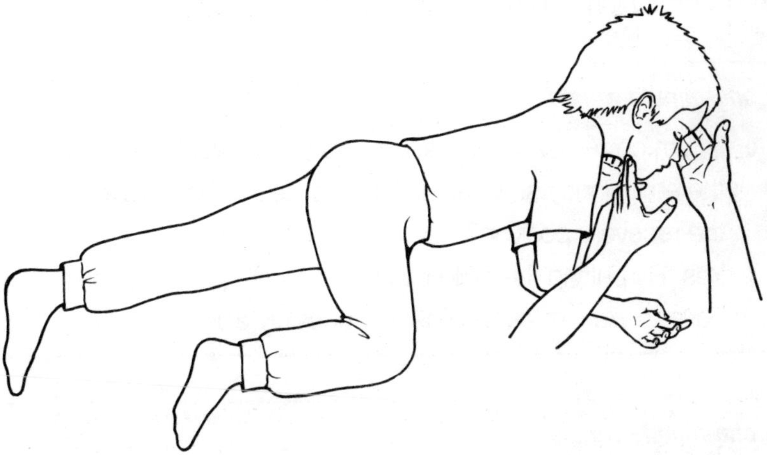

Fig 2 The recovery position

If the child is laying on his back, place him in the recovery position as follows. Kneel beside the child and straighten his legs out, remove any bulky objects from his pockets and remove his spectacles. Then place the child's arm closest to you at a right angle to the child's body. Bring the child's far arm across his chest, then hold his hand, palm outwards, against his cheek. With your other hand, clasp the child's knee furthest from you and pull the leg upward until the foot rests on the floor.

Support the child's head with one hand while pulling the far leg towards you, rolling him onto his side. Tilt the head back to make sure the airway remains open. Continue to monitor the child's breathing and condition, until help arrives.

one-minute wonder

Q If I am on my own and need to go to the telephone to call the emergency services, is it safe to leave the child in the recovery position?

A Yes. By putting the child into the recovery position, you have made him as safe as you possibly can.

one-minute wonder

Q Can a child really 'swallow the tongue' and choke to death?

A Yes, however the term 'swallow the tongue' is used to describe the tongue falling to the back of the throat and blocking the child's airway.

rescue breathing

If you find a child unconscious and he is not breathing, the only way to keep him alive is by getting oxygen into his lungs. This can be done by you breathing for him, a procedure known as rescue breathing. This procedure is often referred to as the 'kiss of life'.

***one-minute** wonder*

Q How do I know how hard to blow while giving rescue breaths?

A We suggest you blow firmly and steadily with just enough force to make the chest visibly rise.

how to carry out rescue breathing

To get your breath into the child's lungs, you must first ensure that his airway is open, as described earlier in this chapter (see page 19). Pinch the child's nose, take a deep breath, place your mouth over the child's mouth and create a good seal. Blow firmly and steadily into the mouth until the child's chest rises (you will see this out of the corner of your eye). If the chest does not rise it is probably because you have not tilted the child's head back far enough. Give a second rescue breath.

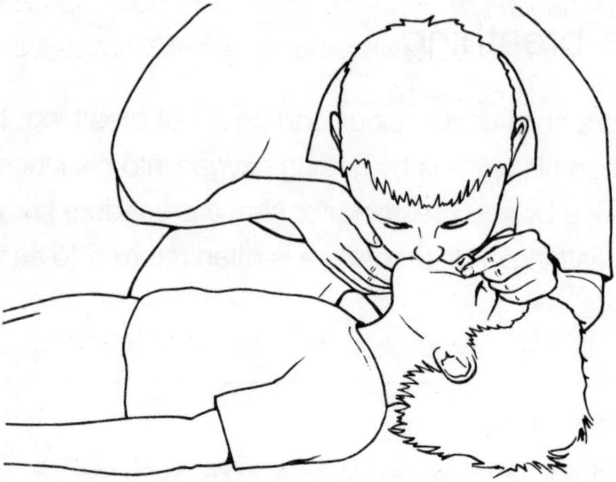

Fig 3 Rescue breathing

Tilt the head back, pinch the nose, place your mouth over the child's mouth and blow.

one-minute wonder

Q What happens if I blow too hard when giving rescue breaths?

A We recommend you blow steadily. This means with just enough force to fill the child's lungs with air, resulting in an upward movement of his chest. If you blow too hard, you will blow air into the stomach and risk the contents of the child's stomach appearing in the mouth.

Once you have given two rescue breaths, you have built up enough oxygen in the child's body, so you must then check if his heart is working otherwise the oxygen will not be circulated around the body by the blood.

how to check circulation

The easiest way to check if the heart is working and blood is being circulated around the body is to look for breathing, coughing or any other obvious movement of the body. Check for up to ten seconds.

If there are signs of circulation, you will have to continue rescue breaths at the rate of 20 breaths per minute.

If there are no signs of circulation, you have to commence CPR. CPR means Cardio Pulmonary Resuscitation. This is the means by which you resuscitate a person who is not breathing and has no signs of circulation. You do this by combining rescue breathing with chest compressions (see page 26). Rescue breathing simulates the work of the lungs and chest compressions simulate the work of the heart.

cardio pulmonary resuscitation (CPR)

To carry out CPR, you must first position your fingers on the child's chest. With the fingers of one hand find the child's lower-most rib. Slide your fingers along the rib to the point where it meets the breastbone. Place the middle finger on this point and the index finger beside it on the breastbone.

Place the heel of your other hand on the lower half of the breastbone next to your fingers. At this point, press down on the chest with the heel of your hand to give chest compressions.

Lean over the child keeping your arms straight. Press down vertically with the heel of your hand to one third of the depth of the child's chest. You should aim to carry out chest compressions at a rate of 100 times per minute.

After giving five compressions, deliver one rescue breath. Continue to deliver cycles of five chest compressions and one rescue breath until either the ambulance arrives, someone else takes over from you, the child moves or starts breathing or you become too exhausted to continue.

If you are alone, it is important that you do one minute of CPR prior to calling for an ambulance.

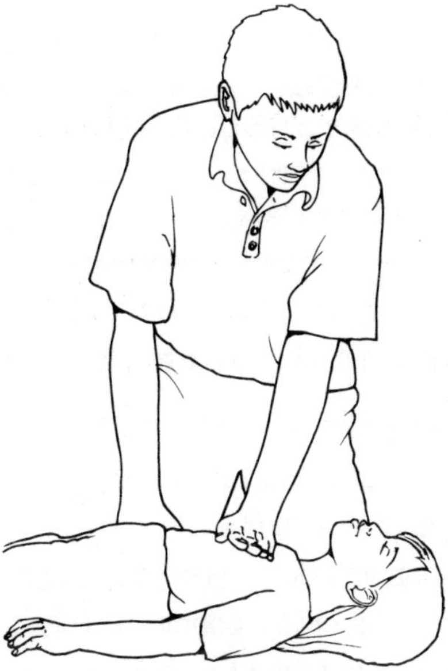

Fig 4 Cardio Pulmonary Resuscitation

Keep your arms straight and use the heel of your hand to press down.

one-minute wonder

Q Carrying out chest compressions at a speed of 100 times per minute seems ridiculously fast. Can you offer any guidance?

A Yes, it is fast. However, clinical evidence tells us that hand position, depth and speed of compression are very important in carrying out CPR. Don't forget that after each five compressions you should deliver one rescue breath.

key skills

On finding a collapsed child with no breathing or signs of circulation, you initially give two rescue breaths followed by five chest compressions, then continue a cycle of one rescue breath followed by five chest compressions.

can CPR really bring a child back to life?

There is much clinical evidence to show that resuscitation (rescue breaths and chest compressions) can keep the main organs of a child alive until an ambulance arrives. It is important to remember that when you do CPR on a child you may not see any obvious change in the child's condition. This does not mean that you are not carrying out the procedure correctly.

one-minute wonder

Q Is it possible for a child to breathe and not to have a heartbeat (circulation)?

A No, it is not possible for this to happen. However, as described earlier in the chapter, it is possible for a child not to breath and have a heartbeat. If this occurs, you just breathe for the child.

summary

If a child is unconscious and breathing, place him in the recovery position. If he is not breathing, do rescue breathing. If he is not breathing and there is no sign of circulation, carry out CPR. Remember to call for an ambulance.

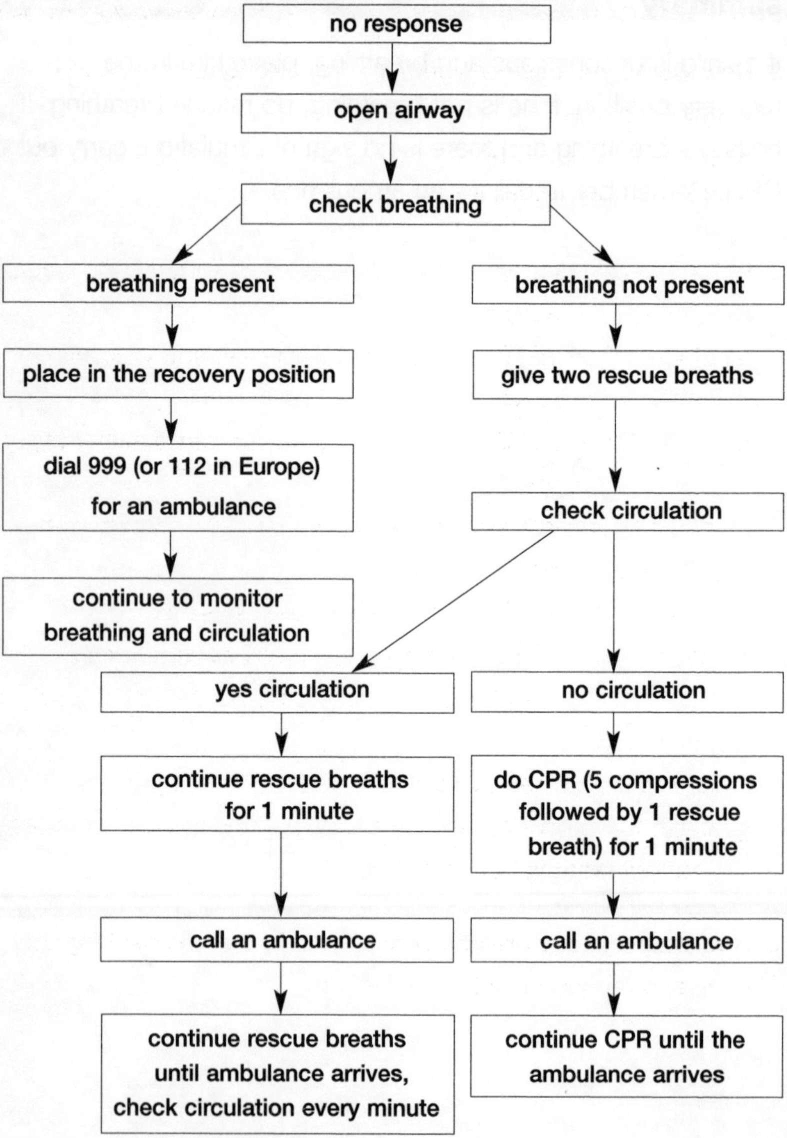

How to respond to an unconscious child

self-testers

1 **How would you assess whether your child is unconscious?**
  a call his name
  b shake him vigorously
  c give him mouth-to-mouth ventilation

2 **Put the following steps in the correct order in which you would perform the recovery position.**
  a place the child's far arm across the chest and hold his hand, palm outwards, against his cheek
  b straighten the child's legs, taking care to remove any bulky objects and spectacles
  c place the child's arm closest to you at right angles, with the elbow bent
  d monitor the child's breathing until help arrives
  e support the child's head with one hand while carefully pulling the far leg towards you and rolling the child onto one side
  f tilt the child's head back to keep the airway open
  g clasp the child's furthest knee, pulling the leg upwards until the foot rests flat on the floor

3 **How many rescue breaths should you do before checking the circulation of your child?**

4 How many rescue breaths and compressions should be given when carrying out CPR on a child?

a three compressions, then one rescue breath

b ten compressions, then two rescue breaths

c five compressions, then one rescue breath

5 At which point on the chest would you perform chest compressions?

---

answers

1 **a**

2 **b**, **c**, **a**, **g**, **e**, **f**, **d**

3 two breaths

4 **c**

5 lower half of the breast bone

3

cuts and scrapes

There are two main types of bleeding: internal and external. External is the most common type of bleeding and it usually results from cuts and scrapes. There are also various types of wounds including abrasions which you probably call grazes – the kind your child may get from falling off his bike – these tend to cover a relatively large area but are not deep. Grazes often contain bits of grit or particles from the ground, and can generally be treated at home. The more severe wounds tend to be incisions caused by sharp objects like knives or blades and, as we know, these are the types of things children like to experiment with. While these tend to be clean cuts, they can be very deep and bleed a lot.

The severity of the wound and the amount of blood lost depends on the size, depth and location of the wound. Lacerations are the type of wounds that have jagged edges – they tend to be tears caused by something that rips rather than cuts the skin. As lacerations are often caused by dirty objects, the risk of infection is high.

There are two types of large blood vessels in the body: veins and arteries. It is their job to carry blood around the body and keep the key organs supplied with oxygen in the blood stream. If a wound results in damage to a vein or artery, this is classified as a severe bleed. The amount of blood lost can be significant and, if not effectively treated, can be life threatening. The presence of a large amount of blood can be terrifying and off-putting for the first person on the scene, and it is very difficult to estimate the amount of blood lost prior to arriving on the scene. When estimating the amount of blood loss, you should take into account the surface on which the blood is falling; a small patch of blood on a deep carpet may signify a larger amount of blood lost than blood covering a large area on a smooth, flat surface. Those of us who have dropped a pint of milk on a tiled kitchen floor appreciate that a small amount of milk can cover a large surface area; the same applies to blood.

cuts and grazes

To treat a minor cut or graze you must sit the child down, gently wash the area using cold running water, and dry the area using a soft pad. Try and remove any pieces of grit that may be embedded in the wound using a soft pad or a very soft brush for this purpose. Then apply pressure on the wound with a pad to stop the bleeding. We do not recommend cotton wool because it is fluffy and may stick to the wound and, as a result, delay the healing. Once the bleeding has stopped, apply a plaster – make sure that the pad of the plaster is large enough to cover the whole of the cut or scrape.

nose bleed

If your child has a nose bleed you should sit him down with his head tilted forward. Pinch the soft part at the end of the nose for ten minutes, discourage your child from sniffing or swallowing and allow any blood in the mouth to drip into a bowl. After ten minutes check if the nose bleed has stopped and clean the child's face. If the nose continues to bleeding after the initial ten-minute pinch, pinch again for another ten minutes. If the bleeding continues for more than half an hour, take the child to hospital.

***one-minute** wonder*

Q Is tilting the head back no longer recommended for the treatment of a nose bleed?

A No. Tilting the head back does not stop the bleeding. If you do this blood can trickle down the back of the throat and make the child feel sick. It can also affect their ability to breathe.

how to treat a severe bleed

The amount of blood a child has in his body depends on his age and size. An older child, for example a seven-year-old child, may have about 5 litres (8 pints) of blood in his body. The effective way to treat a severe bleed is by placing pressure directly on the wound. You, as the first aider, can do this or you can encourage the child to do it if he is sufficiently brave. Once you have applied pressure to the wound, raise the injured limb or part of the body above the level of the child's heart. Once you have done this, lay the child down with the head low, ensure that he is comfortable, and keep pressing on the wound for up to ten minutes. Your aim is to stem the blood flow and allow the clotting process to begin – this is the body's way of stopping the blood escaping.

Once you have stemmed the blood flow with pressure, cover the wound with a dressing and bandage. Ensure that the bandage is not too tight as it could cut off the blood supply. If the blood comes through the first bandage, do not remove it. Apply another bandage on top. If blood continues to seep through the two dressing pads you must then, and only then, remove both pads and replace with a new one. If there is an object embedded in the wound, do not try and remove it as this may cause further bleeding. We recommend that you use two rolls of padding (as in dressing pads), placing them on each side of the wound.

Ensure pressure is placed on the side of the wound, not pressing on the object itself, and bandage over the object.

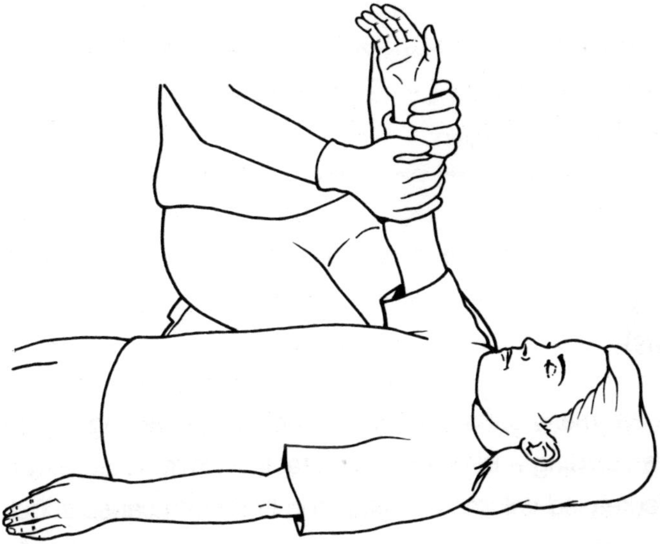

Fig 5 Treating a severe bleed

Once this treatment has been applied, you should continue to support the injury and reassure the child, and then arrange for him to be taken to hospital for further assessment.

key skills

Place direct pressure on the wound and elevate the injured area above the level of the heart. Cover the wound with a dressing and arrange for the child to be taken to hospital.

one-minute wonder

Q If blood comes through the dressing, why do you suggest leaving it in place rather than removing it?

A If you remove the dressing, you could dislodge the blood clots that were forming underneath and the wound could start bleeding again.

shock

There are many causes of shock, including bleeding, burns, severe vomiting and diarrhoea. In fact, anything that results in the decreased volume of fluid in the body can cause shock. Other types of shock can result from head injuries, and allergic conditions commonly known as an anaphylactic shock. In Chapter 5 we describe in some detail how to recognize and treat anaphylactic shock, which is an extreme allergic reaction to something that has been taken into the body.

The term 'shock' tends to be misused in our everyday language; many people tend to use it to describe an emotional response to something they've seen or heard. For example,

'I went into shock when I found out I had won the lottery' is not the type of shock we are talking about in this chapter. Here, we are talking about clinical shock, a condition where the body responds in a particular way to an injury or illness.

Blood loss is one of the most common causes of shock in children. Shock occurs when there is an inadequate supply of blood, for whatever reason, reaching the key organs in the body. The more blood a child loses, the greater the level of shock. It is difficult to provide an accurate guide to how a child's body will respond to blood loss because this very much depends on the age and size of the child. The following guidance is based on the average child.

If your child loses 0.25 litres of blood (½ pint), there is little or no effect on the child's body. If the child loses twice this amount, the signs of shock become evident. You will notice that the pulse rate increases, the skin will appear cold, clammy and sweaty, the child will appear weak and dizzy, feel sick and complain of feeling thirsty. As the shock develops, the child will become confused and begin gasping for air (also known as goldfish breathing). If the condition goes untreated, the child will fall unconscious and may require resuscitation. It is vitally important that if your child is going into shock you should follow the instructions given overleaf.

treatment of shock

If your child goes into shock, you must:

- lay him down
- raise and support his legs on a cushion or pile of blankets
- loosen any tight clothing around the child
- keep him warm.

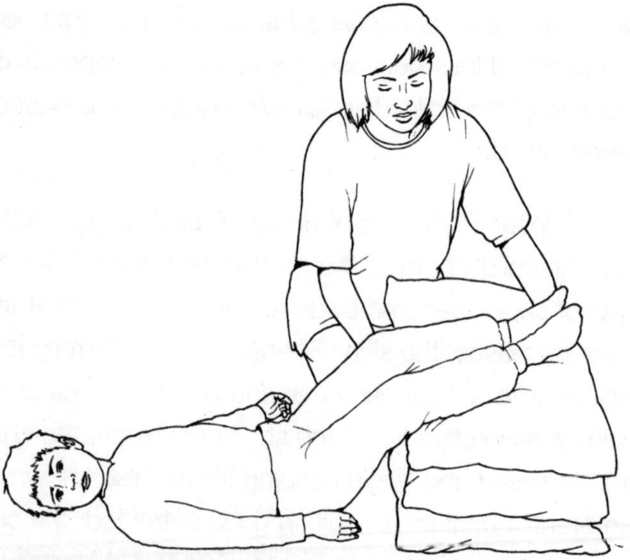

Fig 6 Treating shock

Remember in the case of shock as a result of bleeding, to also keep the injured limb elevated. This and raising the legs results in a greater level of circulation in the body by moving the blood which is in the legs up to the key organs that need it. It is also important to reassure the child. Talk to the child, keep him warm, and monitor him closely until the ambulance arrives. Some suggest that the best treatment for shock is a cup of sweet tea or a drink of alcohol. We do not recommend that the child has anything to eat or drink and certainly not alcohol. If he complains of thirst, moisten his lips with some water.

key skills

If you child goes into shock, lay him down, raise his legs, keep him warm and call an ambulance.

5 • 5

internal bleeding

The term 'internal bleeding' is used to describe bleeding inside the body which is not always evident when you look at the child. Any sign of blood loss from a body orifice should be taken seriously because it may indicate internal bleeding. Orifices include ears, nose, mouth, anus, urethra and vagina.

Internal bleeding can occur as a result of an earlier injury or may result from a fracture. Injury to some of the large organs housed in the abdomen, including the spleen, may result in internal bleeding that can only be recognized by bruising, hardness and tenderness of the abdomen.

If you suspect internal bleeding, you should make the child as comfortable as possible, treat for shock if necessary, and call for an ambulance.

one-minute wonder

Q Is fainting a form of shock?

A Fainting is a temporary loss of consciousness caused by a reduction of blood supply to the brain. To treat a faint you should ensure that the child has plenty of fresh air, and raise his legs. He usually recovers very quickly.

summary

Cuts and scrapes are very common injuries in childhood and if there is a lot of bleeding the sight of the blood can be frightening for everyone concerned. It is important to stay calm and focus on applying pressure to the wound, raising the limb and watching for shock.

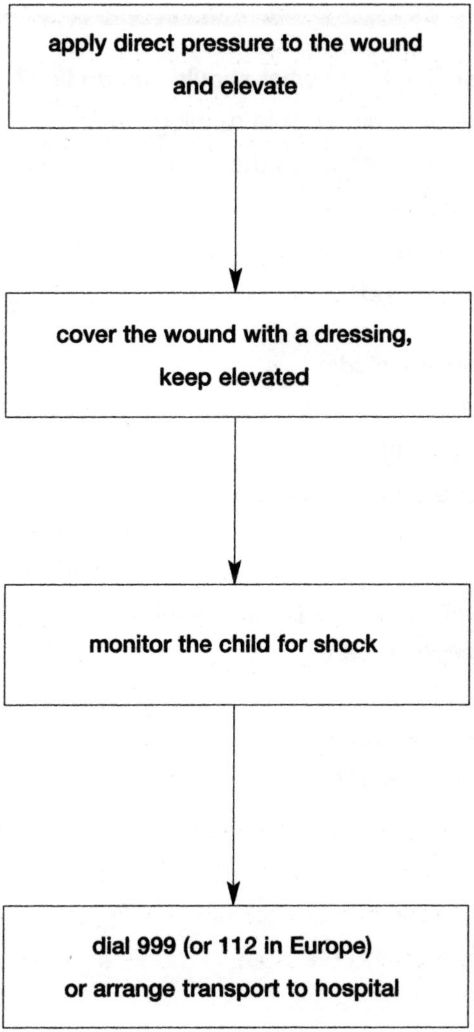

How to treat a severe bleed

self-testers

1 To treat a severe bleed what should you do first?

a place the area under cold running water

b apply direct pressure to the wound and raise it above the level of the heart

c lie the child flat

d clean the wound

2 Signs of shock include:

a pale skin

b slow breathing

c floppiness and drowsiness

d fast pulse

3 To clean a small wound you can use:

a an antiseptic cream

b a soft pad

c a piece of cotton wool

d cold running water

---

answers

1 **b**

2 **a**, **c** and **d**

3 **b** and **d**

4

how to deal with choking

Children have a tendency to put objects in their mouths, talk at mealtimes and to not chew their food properly. They also like to put small toys, pen tops, or any other objects that you leave lying around in their mouths. This, in addition to their liking for boiled sweets or lollipops, puts children at risk of choking on something. The seriousness of a choking incident is dependent on the size and shape of the object. For example, a small round, smooth shape like a marble can be dislodged more easily than an object with rough and sharp edges like a building brick. If the offending object blocks a significant part of the airway and the child stops breathing, it is crucial to try and dislodge it as quickly as possible. Remember that choking can be extremely distressing, it is therefore important that you try and remain calm, and that you reassure the child while carrying out the care outlined overleaf.

how to treat choking

It may be obvious to you if your child is choking; he may be clutching his throat and have difficulty in breathing while unable to speak. You should check in the child's mouth to see if you can see the offending object. If so, remove it. Do not blindly put your fingers in a child's mouth. If you cannot see the object, encourage the child to cough. If this does not dislodge it, bend the child forwards and give up to five sharp slaps between his shoulder blades (see Figure 7).

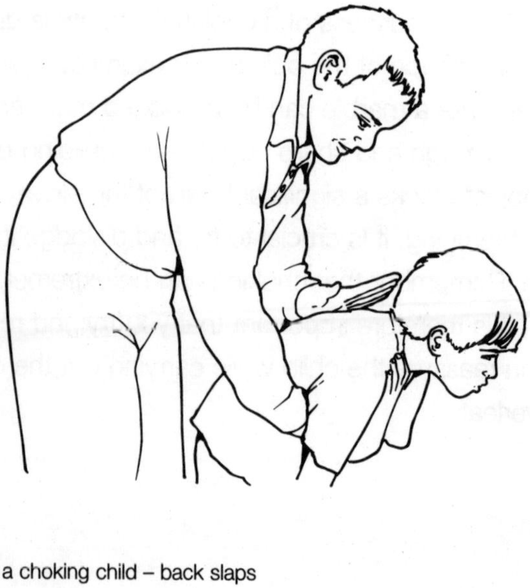

Fig 7 Treating a choking child – back slaps

Check in the mouth again. If back slaps have not worked, you should carry out chest thrusts. Stand or kneel behind the child, make a fist and place it over the lower part of the child's breastbone (see Figure 8). Hold the fist with your other hand and pull inwards up to five times. Leave a two-second gap between each chest thrust. Pressing on the bottom of the child's breastbone causes an artificial cough. This may be enough to move the object. Once the cycle of the chest thrusts is complete, check in the mouth.

Fig 8 Treating a choking child – chest thrusts

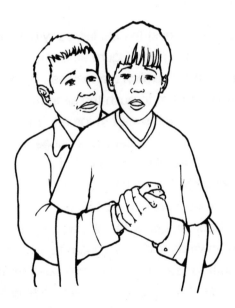

one-minute wonder

Q Why do you advise against putting your finger into the child's mouth unless you can see the object?

A You should not put your finger into the mouth of a child unless you can see the object because otherwise you could push the object further down the throat or damage the soft tissue at the back of the mouth which is extremely sensitive.

If the back slaps and chest thrusts fail, carry out a procedure called abdominal thrusts (see Figure 9). Some people refer to this procedure as the 'Heimlich manoeuvre'. By pressing on the child's abdomen, you aim to push the air from the lungs up through the windpipe with sufficient force to move the blockage. We are often asked if this procedure is dangerous and uncomfortable for the child. It can be, but it is also effective in treating a choking child when back slaps and chest thrusts have failed. Stand or kneel behind the child, place your fists in the middle of his abdomen below the rib cage, hold your other hand over it and pull inwards and upwards up to five times. Check in the child's mouth to see if the object has been moved. Once you have carried out this procedure, even if the child recovers, we suggest that you seek medical advice to check whether there is any internal damage.

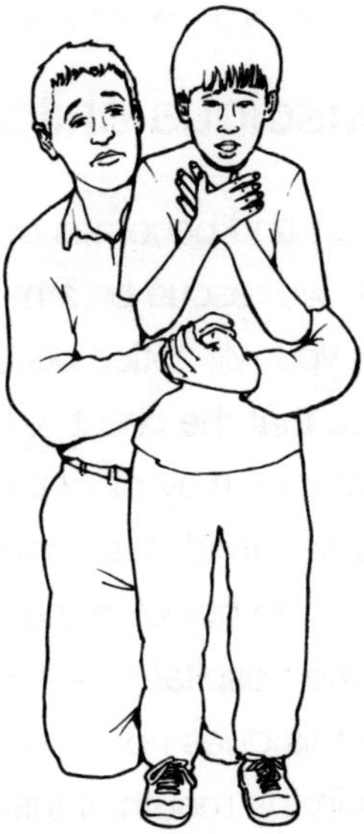

Fig 9 Treating a choking child – abdominal thrusts

If the object has not moved, continue the cycle of five back slaps followed by five chest thrusts and abdominal thrusts three times and then call for an ambulance. Continue the cycle until the ambulance arrives or the object becomes dislodged. At any point there is the possibility that the child may stop breathing. Be prepared to resuscitate.

a choking, unconscious child

If your child stops breathing and becomes unconscious because of choking you must give two rescue breaths. If air will not go in because of the blockage, you will notice because you will feel resistance and you will see that the chest will not rise. Some people are concerned that they may blow the object into the child's lungs. While this is not an ideal situation, at least the child will be able to breathe, and the object in the lung can be dealt with on his admission to the hospital. Make four further attempts to get air into his lungs. If this does not work, give five chest compressions and check in the mouth. If this has not worked, give one rescue breath and five chest compressions for a minute (see Chapter 2, page 23–27). Call for an ambulance if you have not done so already. Continue one rescue breath and five chest compressions until the ambulance arrives or your child begins to breathe for himself.

key skills

If a child is choking and conscious:

- get him to cough
- check in his mouth to see if the object has moved
- give up to five back slaps
- check his mouth
- give up to five chest thrusts
- check his mouth
- give up to five abdominal thrusts
- check his mouth

eyes and ears

In addition to placing items in the mouth, children often get foreign objects in their eyes or ears. In terms of the eye, this is most commonly a piece of grit or dirt. If something is embedded in the eye or is sticking to the eye, you should not attempt to remove it. Cover the injured eye with a sterile pad and take the child to hospital for medical treatment. If the object is floating around the eye, you should first sit the child down. Look at the whole eye while separating the eyelids. If you can see the offending object, wash it out using water. Tilt the child's head to one side and, ideally using a jug of water, aim the water to the corner of the eye. This ensures that the whole eye will be cleaned. You can use a small receptacle to catch the water. If this does not remove the object, you can use the corner of a damp handkerchief or pad to lift the object clear of the eye.

If the object is not immediately visible, check under the eyelid. You can ask your child to assist you by lifting the eyelid up. It is important to remember that your child may continue to experience some discomfort in the eye for a little while after the object has been removed. If you are concerned that the eye is not fully clean, seek medical advice.

If your child places something in his ear canal, it important to ascertain as quickly and as early as possible what the object is. If, on inspecting the ear, the object is visible, we do not recommend that you try and remove it as this may cause pain and may damage the eardrum. Reassure the child and take him to hospital for medical advice.

Children have also been known to put foreign objects in their nose. If you suspect that this has occurred, inspect the nose. Also note that the child may have some difficulty in breathing. There may be some injury to the nose resulting in swelling or there may be evidence of blood. It is important that you reassure the child, encouraging him to breathe through his mouth. Take the child to hospital. As with any object in the ear, do not attempt to remove it, even if it's visible.

In the unfortunate event of an insect getting into your child's ear, you should sit the child down and tilt the head to one side with the affected ear upper most. Then pour tepid water into the ear until the insect floats out. If it is not possible to remove the insect in this way take the child to hospital.

summary

Choking can be very scary, therefore it is import to remain calm and reassure the child, ensure the back slaps are firm and never place your fingers blindly in the mouth of a child. If the child is conscious, remember back slaps followed by chest thrusts followed by abdominal thrusts.

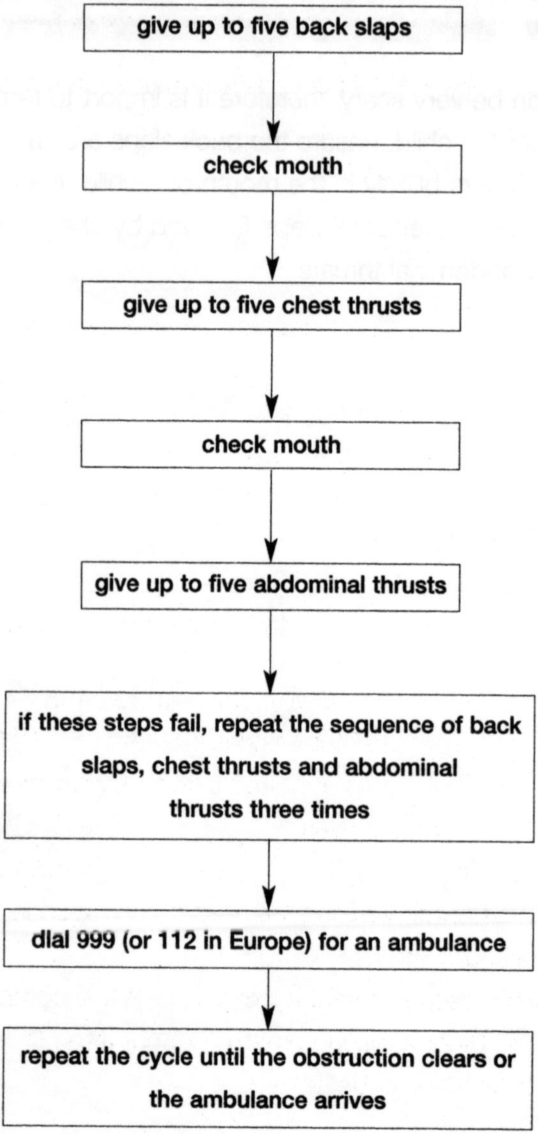

How to treat a choking child

self-testers

1 If you discover your child is choking what is the first thing you should do?

a give five sharp back slaps
b encourage him to cough
c give chest thrusts

2 What is the correct procedure for a choking child who is conscious?

a five back slaps followed by five chest thrusts. Repeat cycle three times then call for an ambulance
b five back slaps, five chest thrusts, five abdominal thrusts. Then call for an ambulance
c five back slaps, five chest thrusts, five abdominal thrusts. Repeat cycle three times then call for an ambulance

3 What should you do if your child stops breathing?

a give two rescue breaths making five attempts. If this fails give five chest compressions followed by two rescue breaths until help arrives
b give two rescue breaths up to five times. If this fails give five chest compressions followed by one rescue breath until help arrives
c give one rescue breath. If this fails give five compressions followed by one rescue breath. Repeat three times and then call for an ambulance

4 If a child places something in his ear what should you do?

a attempt to remove it using tweezers

b tilt the head to one side and try and shake it out

c do not try and remove it and take the child to hospital

d put a dressing over the ear

answers

1 b

2 c

3 a

4 c

5

bites, stings, bleach and berries

In this chapter we will look at the most common types of poison and how they enter and affect the body. You should remember that poisons can be swallowed, inhaled, injected or are the result of bites and stings. All of these poisons require a different type of consideration and treatment. The number of incidents involving any type of poison can be significantly reduced by taking some simple precautions in the home and outdoors.

insect bites and stings

The most common insect stings are from wasps, bees and hornets. These tend to be more painful than dangerous. However, there has been much recent publicity about the extreme allergic reaction a very small number of people have to insect stings. The risk of such a reaction is increased if your child is stung in the mouth or throat, or suffers from multiple stings. It is possible to reduce the risk of your child being bitten or stung by using insect repellent and dressing him in long-sleeved t-shirts and long trousers.

insect bites

Insects that bite rather than sting include midges, flies and bedbugs. However, these bites are not serious and generally result in localized itchiness, minor swelling, redness of the skin and small bumps, and they fade quite quickly. These require little first aid and are generally treated by keeping the skin cool and dry, and by the application of creams recommended by your pharmacist. It is very rare for insect bites to result in an allergic reaction.

insect stings

It is usually obvious to a parent or a carer if their child has been stung by a wasp, bee or other insect. The child will cry as a result of the pain and you will notice redness and swelling at the site of the sting. Also, some insects leave their sting in the skin. If this happens, you should scrape the sting off the skin using a flat object; a credit card is ideal. We suggest the sting be scraped off the skin rather than pulled out using tweezers or a similar tool. The reason for this is the actual sting itself contains poison and if it is squeezed rather than brushed or scraped away, it may result in more poison being injected into the skin.

One you have removed the sting, apply a cold compress to the affected area. You can use a bag of frozen vegetables for this purpose; peas, sweetcorn or small vegetables are best as they mould around the injury more easily. Leave the cold compress in place for up to ten minutes. Reassure the child throughout the treatment.

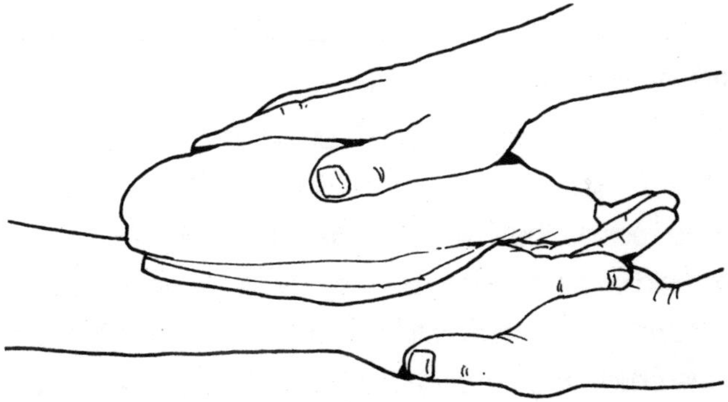

Fig 10 Applying a cold compress

All children will have some type of allergic reaction to a sting because the sting contains poison and it will go into the child's body. In a small minority of cases, a child can have a severe allergic reaction resulting in red blotchy skin, swelling around the face and neck and difficulty in breathing. If this occurs, call an ambulance and be prepared to resuscitate your child if necessary (see Chapter 2).

key skills

To treat an insect sting, the most common of these being wasp or bee stings, check the site for redness or swelling. Remove the sting if it is in the skin and place a cold compress on the affected site.

---

one-minute wonder

Q How do I treat a sting to the mouth? Should I put ice in my child's mouth?

A No, to reduce the pain or swelling in the child's mouth, give him cold water to drink. Be very careful, when examining the child's mouth for a sting, that you don't touch the back of the child's mouth because it is very sensitive to touch and may swell.

one-minute wonder

Q Is there a risk of causing damage by placing ice on a child's skin?

A A cold burn can result if you place ice directly on the skin. Our advice is that you cover the ice pack first with a tea towel or similar and only leave it in place for ten minutes.

poisons

We referred earlier to an insect sting containing poison. However, we more commonly associate poisoning with something a child has found under the sink and decided to drink, or tablets or medicines that look like sweets. It is also important to remember that poisons can be inhaled, for example, smoke and fumes from cleaning products and products used in the garden. Finally, there is food poisoning.

Clearly, many incidents involving poisons can be avoided if appropriate precautions are taken. Our advice is to assume that all cleaning products are potentially poisonous; keep them locked away or out of reach of children. If you are visiting another house, you can subtly check if it is child-friendly and whether there are any poisonous substances within reach. Many poisonous products offer specific advice on the label about how to treat accidental swallowing of the contents, and some have a number you can call for advice. Always follow the manufacturer's guidance for use and, in terms of food poisoning, take precautions when preparing and storing food. It is important to remember that young children may on occasion like to sample the pet foods that they find on the floor. While this may not be dangerous to your child in small quantities, because of the immaturity of their digestive systems it may result in vomiting and diarrhoea. If you think your child has eaten some pet food, seek medical advice.

In this part of the book, we will only look at poisons that your child may swallow or inhale. Poisons are often referred to as 'toxic' or 'non toxic'. There is another category of poisons we have referred to as 'potentially toxic'. We recognize that the manufacturers have made great efforts to ensure that their products are not accidently swallowed, including the introduction of child-resistant caps, yet some children seem to manage to open these. The most important piece of advice we can give is to never put poisons into other bottles – especially soft-drink bottles.

non toxic

Non-toxic substances that will not, in small quantities, present a risk to your child include:

- pencils
- crayons
- water-based glue
- blue tack
- bath oil
- lipstick.

If your child shows some reaction to swallowing these or has taken a large quantity, seek medical advice.

potentially toxic

Items under this heading include:

- detergents
- bleach
- disinfectants
- nail varnish remover
- toilet cleaning blocks.

Yes, to some children the toilet cleaning black that sits under your toilet rim smells nice and is an appealing colour. Our advice is to always seek medical advice if your child has taken any of these.

toxic

If your child has taken any of the following, you should call for an ambulance immediately:

- anti freeze
- oven cleaner
- dishwashing powder, tablets or liquid
- herbicides
- insecticides
- petrol or petrol derivatives.

bleach and chemicals

If a child has swallowed chemicals, you may notice some around his mouth or be able to smell it on his breath. Some bleach will cause burning around the mouth and lips, and possible discoloration of the lips. If you suspect this has happened, wipe away any excess from the skin, give the child sips of water or milk to drink (do not make the child vomit). Find out what the chemical was and seek medical advice. If you need to take the child for hospital treatment, take the suspected bottle of chemical with you.

one-minute wonder

Q I thought you should make the child vomit, as this would get the poison out of his body.

A No, we do not advise that you make your child vomit if he has swallowed a corrosive poison. This is because vomitting may make the condition worse by damaging the stomach and the tubes that carry food to the stomach. If it burned when it went down it will burn again as it comes up.

drug poisoning

Children are attracted to tablets and medicines, and can mistake them for sweets or fruit juice. If you suspect your child has swallowed drugs, you should try and find out what he has taken and in what quantity. Seek medical advice immediately. Do not make the child vomit or give him anything to drink until you have received medical advice.

***one-minute* wonder**

Q How can I accurately guess how many tablets my child has swallowed?

A Count the number of tablets remaining in the container and try and base your guess on how many were in there originally. Use the same approach if the medicine is in liquid form.

***one-minute* wonder**

Q Why should I not give the child anything to drink until I have sought medical advice?

A If your child has swallowed tablets, fluids will dissolve them more quickly in his stomach and this means the drug will enter his bloodstream more quickly. In some cases, this could put the child at greater risk.

***one-minute* wonder**

Q If my child vomits after swallowing some tablets, I was told you should not throw this away.

A You can collect a small amount of the child's vomit to take to the doctor or hospital with you. This can be helpful in aiding medical staff to analyse the poison and administer the correct treatment.

plants and berries

If you suspect a child may have swallowed a poisonous plant, flower or berries, try to find out what he has eaten, and look around his mouth and inside it to see if any pieces remain. Do not make the child sick. Seek medical advice. If you have to go to the doctor, have a sample of the plant or berries with you. Likewise, if the child vomits take a sample with you. Check your home for pot plants that may be poisonous if swallowed, and take precautions if visiting parks or garden centres.

one-minute wonder

Q My child reached out of his buggy when we were on a country walk, and he was stung on the hand and arms by nettles. What should I have done?

A Nettle rash can be painful and itchy. Thankfully, these symptoms only last a short time. Place a cold compress on the area or soothe the area with calamine lotion.

food poisoning

The most common signs and symptoms of food poisoning are diarrhoea and vomiting. A child suffering from episodes of vomiting or episodes of diarrhoea can become dehydrated.

Your aim is to replace lost fluids by giving the child cooled boiled water, or a rehydratring solution like Dioralyte. Seek medical advice.

key skills

The principles for the treatment of poisoning are as follows:

- find out what the child took
- at what time did he take it?
- how much did he swallow?
- reassure the child
- seek medical advice.

animal bites

In the event of your child being bitten by an animal, wash the wound thoroughly using soap and warm water. Rinse the wound under water for at least five minutes to wash away any dirt or residue. Once you have done this, clean and dry the wound using a pad or tissue, and cover it using a small dressing or a plaster. It is also worth remembering that your child should be protected against tetanus infection. Therefore, please ensure that your child's tetanus vaccination is current and up to date and, if not, make arrangements to see your doctor.

If the animal bite results in a large wound, follow the advice on bleeding given in Chapter 3. If your child has been bitten while abroad, remember that he might need an anti-rabies injection.

summary

While we do everything we can to make our homes and gardens child friendly, it is not possible to make them accident-proof. However, some precautions are more straightforward than others, the key one being the storage of poisons – keep them out of reach. Protect your child against stings and bites by using repellent and appropriate clothing. If in doubt about what your child has swallowed or been stung by, seek medical advice.

self-testers

1 What should you use to remove a sting?

a tweezers

b a thumbnail

c a needle

d a credit card

2 If you think your child has swallowed a toxic substance what should you do first?

a call an ambulance

b try to make him vomit

c give hot milk

d give sips of water

3 Which of the following is potentially toxic for your child?

a lipstick

b bleach

c crayons

d nail varnish remover

4 How should you treat a sting in the mouth?

a put ice on his tongue

b give a hot drink

c apply a cold compress to the mouth

d give cold water to drink

---

answers

1 **b** and **d**

2 **a**

3 **b** and **d**

4 **d**

6

burns and blisters

In our research we have found that burns and scalds are some of the most common injuries affecting children, and they are also the ones that commonly receive incorrect first-aid treatment. When treating a burn or scald, the aims are to cool the area quickly, thus relieving the pain, and to minimize the risk of infection.

We use the term 'burn' to describe an injury that occurs from direct contact with heat or flame. 'Scalds' tend to be caused by liquid or steam.

In the case of children, it is very important that you act quickly when treating a burn. If you do not, the skin and underlying tissue will continue to burn and this will result in your child being in considerable pain. The burn will become more severe and, ultimately, this will result in more scarring of the skin.

how to treat a burn

The most effective way to treat a burn or scald is to place the affected area under cold running water for at least ten minutes (Figure 11). In treating young children, it is important not to immerse their whole body in water as this may cause hypothermia. If you do not have cold running water, you can place the burnt area in a bowl of water. However, this is not as effective as running water. If cold water is not available, you can use milk or a non-fizzy soft drink. You can use a shower to cool a large burnt area, but you must always ensure the shower is on a cold setting and the water pressure is low. Warm or high pressure water will only make the condition worse. We do not recommend creams or ointments as part of the initial treatment because they are not very effective unless the area is first cooled. Furthermore, if creams are applied they may have to be removed once the child arrives in hospital to enable medical staff to assess the burn.

Burns to the mouth or throat can be potentially life threatening because swelling in this area can affect a child's breathing. You will need to act very quickly. If this occurs, call for an ambulance, loosen all clothing around the child's neck and be prepared to resuscitate (see Chapter 2).

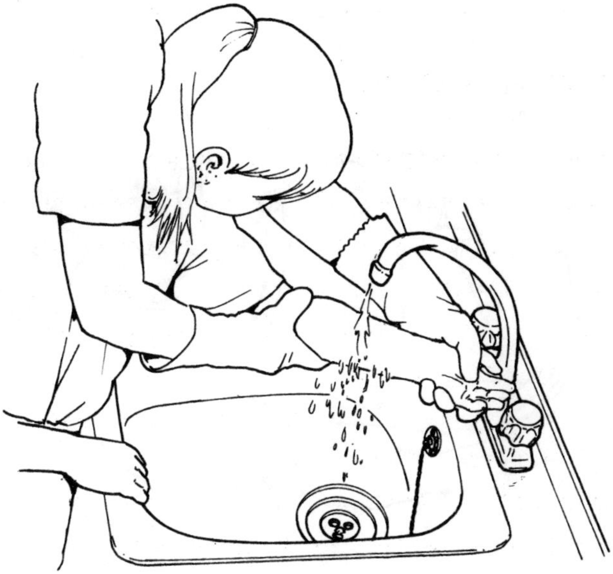

Fig 11 Cooling a burn

It is common for swelling to occur following a burn. Therefore, it is important to remove any tight clothing before the swelling occurs. It is possible to remove clothing while the burn is being cooled. Do not remove any clothing or material that may be sticking to a burn.

Fig 12 Covering a burn

Once the area has been cooled, you should cover the burn with a clean, non-fluffy material. This will help to prevent the wound becoming infected and it will reduce the pain. An alternative dressing for a burn is a clean plastic bag (freezer/sandwich bag), or clean cling film. A bag is particularly useful for treating burns to the hand and lower arm. Place the bag over the hand or arm and secure it in place using a plaster or bandage. Cling film is best for arms or legs. Discard the first piece of film as it may be contaminated by touch or food. Place a clean piece of cling film loosely around the burn. When the burn is cooled and covered, seek medical advice.

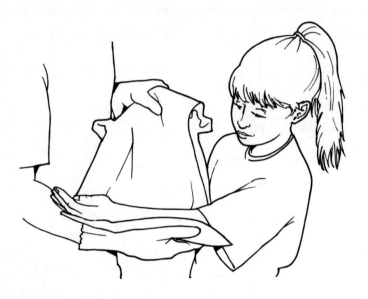

In a very small number of cases a severe burn over a large area may result in the child going into shock (see page 38).

key skills

To treat a burn or a scald, place it under cold running water for at least ten minutes. Cover the burn and seek medical advice if necessary.

blisters

Blisters often require little treatment as the fluid that is contained within them is reabsorbed back into the skin. However, if they do burst you should apply a clean dressing to the affected area. This will reduce the risk of infection. This advice applies whether the blister results from contact with heat or friction, for example, your child wearing ill-fitting shoes.

one-minute wonder

Q When blisters appear on the skin after a scald, should you burst them?

A No, you should avoid touching the burn or bursting blisters because doing this increases the risk of infection and delays the healing process.

summary

When treating a burn or scald act quickly but try and stay calm. Do not remove the child's clothing if it is stuck to the skin or if removing the clothing will result in a delay in cooling the affected area. As part of your first-aid treatment it is not advisable to burst blisters as this may increase the risk of infection.

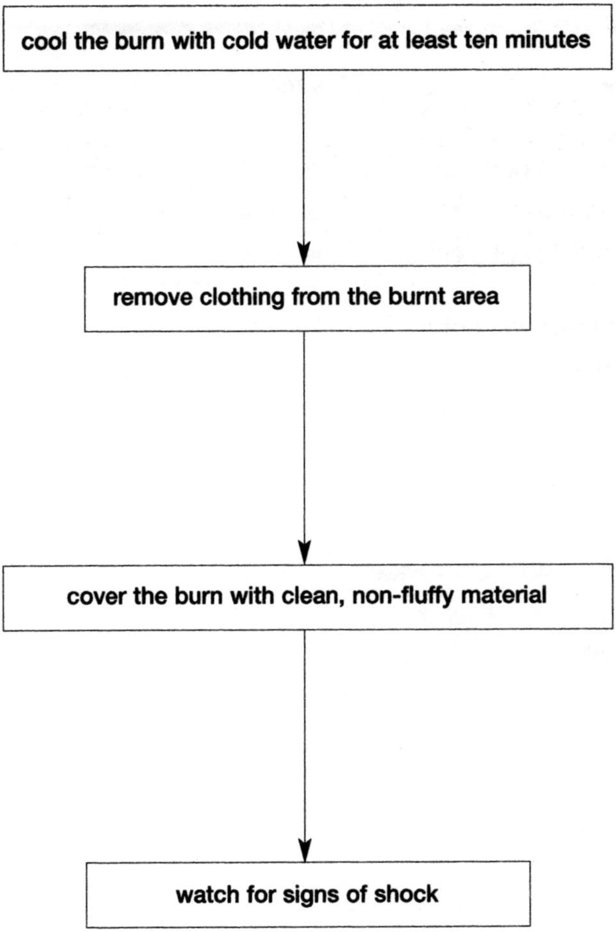

cool the burn with cold water for at least ten minutes
remove clothing from the burnt area
cover the burn with clean, non-fluffy material
watch for signs of shock

How to deal with burns and blisters

self-testers

1 In the event of a burn, what is the first thing you should do?

- **a** call an ambulance
- **b** cool the burn for ten minutes with cold water
- **c** put a piece of cling film around the burn
- **d** put antiseptic cream on the burn

2 What must you not do if a child is burnt?

- **a** place him in a cold bath
- **b** apply an antiseptic cream
- **c** place the burn in a bowl of cool water

3 To treat a burst blister you should:

- **a** run it under cold water
- **b** apply an antiseptic cream
- **c** apply a clean dressing

answers

1 **b**

2 **a** and **b**

3 **c**

7

sprains, strains and broken bones

Injuries to bones, muscles and joints remain the most common injuries suffered by children. A child' s bone is very different to an adult's because the child's bone is still growing, and injuries to joints and muscles are often due to a child's energetic nature. It is often difficult for the person delivering first aid to be able to differentiate between a sprain, a strain or, on occasions, a broken bone.

how to treat a strain or sprain

sprains

Injuries that occur as a result of the pulling or stretching of a joint are described as a sprain, and it is often only the location of the injury that differentiates it from a strain. Sprains occur at joints and involve ligaments. The most common site for a sprain is the ankle. The cause of the injury may often indicate what type of injury you are dealing with. For example, did your child strike a hard object? Was his ankle or wrist twisted? Your aim is to reduce the swelling at the site of the injury, and this will often result in a reduction in the pain and discomfort felt by your child. On inspecting the site of the injury you may notice that there is tenderness, and it may appear warm to touch. There may be some evidence of swelling or bruising. To effectively treat a sprain, you should use the RICE procedure:

- **R**est the injured part
- **I**ce – apply ice or a cold pad to the injured area
- **C**ompress the injury using a bandage and soft padding
- **E**levate the injured part.

strains

A strain is an injury to muscle or tendons and tends to occur when the muscle is stretched, for instance, when playing sport. The signs and symptoms are similar to those of a sprain, however there may be more evidence of bruising due to the fact that a muscle is involved. Your initial treatment is the same as the treatment described for a strain – use RICE.

Once this treatment has been applied, the level of discomfort should reduce and the child should begin to feel better. If you suspect there may be an underlying fracture, seek medical advice.

one-minute wonder

Q You recommend a cold compress as part of the treatment for a sprain and strain. My friend is a physiotherapist and she suggests a hot compress. Which is it?

A A cold compress is part of the initial treatment to reduce the immediate pain and swelling; other health-care professionals use a warm compress as part of the ongoing treatment.

Rest the injured area by getting the child to lay down or sit down. If the ankle is involved, discourage him from walking on it in the initial stages of the treatment. Then cool the area with an ice pack or frozen vegetables; do not apply the cold pack directly onto the skin but wrap it in a tea towel or similar. If ice is not available, use a cold flannel or towel. You should then bandage the injury site by first placing a thick layer of cotton wool around the injury and then bandaging over the cotton wool. Once the bandage is in place, check the child's circulation every ten minutes to ensure the bandage is not restricting the blood flow to the limb beyond the injury. Finally, elevate the limb by placing it on a chair or any other object. If nothing else is available ask a bystander to support it in a comfortable position. Keeping the limb elevated helps to reduce the swelling and the pain. If in doubt, seek medical advice.

key skills

Use the RICE procedure as the initial treatment for a strain or sprain.

fractures

We use the term 'fracture' to describe a break or a crack in a bone. There are various types of fractures but they tend to fall into two main categories – open and closed fractures. In an open fracture the skin is broken at the site of the fracture, and in a closed fracture there is no break in the surface of the skin. Fractures tend to result from direct or indirect force on the body. For example, direct force happens if a car hits the child, and indirect force results from the twisting or wrenching of a bone.

It is very difficult for the first aider to differentiate between a sprain, strain or a closed fracture. This is further complicated in young children where there is a type of closed fracture known as a 'greenstick fracture'. This is where the bone doesn't actually break, rather it bends like a green stick, hence the name.

The signs and symptoms of a fracture include pain, bruising and swelling at the fracture site. The pain level tends to increase significantly if the injured part is moved. The limb may be in an unnatural position and, in the case of an open fracture, the bone ends may be protruding through the skin.

Your aim when treating a fracture is to prevent avoidable movement at the site of the injury and, in the case of an open fracture, take precautions to avoid the wound or the bone becoming infected. Try and avoid any action that causes further damage, especially in the case of an open fracture where there is a risk of further damage to the tissue or underlying blood vessels. In the case of treating fractures, less movement means less pain. All suspected fractures require assessment in hospital. You can transport the child yourself or, for more serious injuries including all open fractures and if you suspect there is more than one fracture or if the child is showing signs of shock, call for an ambulance. Do not give the child anything to eat or drink as this may delay hospital treatment. Be prepared to treat for shock (see Chapter 3, page 38).

key skills

If you suspect a fracture, avoid moving the affected area as much as possible. If the child has an open fracture or appears to be going into shock, call for an ambulance.

one-minute wonder

Q Is it true that a fracture is not as painful as a sprain?

A Both fractures and sprains can be painful, but a lot depends on the site of the injury and the pain threshold of the injured child. We do not think it is possible to give a definitive answer about which is the most painful.

closed fractures

If you suspect a closed fracture, you should try to prevent movement at the site of the injury because movement increases the pain and may cause further damage. Then make arrangements for the child to be taken to hospital. Closed fractures can include a broken leg, a broken foot, a broken collarbone, a broken arm, a broken hand and broken fingers.

broken leg

In the case of a broken leg, advise the child to lay as still as possible. Call for an ambulance. Reassure him and support the leg above and below the fracture site.

broken foot

In children, this injury usually results from the foot being crushed. You should use the RICE procedure and arrange for the child to be taken to hospital.

broken collarbone

This injury commonly occurs as a result of indirect force. For example, a child falling from his bicycle will often put his arms out to protect himself; this force then travels up the arm to the neck and shoulder area. You can recognize a broken collarbone as there will be increased pain and tenderness in the area of the neck and shoulder. The child will be very protective of the injured site and may turn his head to the side of the injury. This can be treated by sitting the child down, getting him to support the injury by placing his arm on the injured side across his chest. Apply an elevation sling (see Figure 13) to the injured side and secure the arm in place with a broad-fold bandage (see Figure 14). Take the child to hospital.

broken arm

The treatment for a fracture of the upper arm, forearm or the wrist is as follows. Ask the child to sit down and advise him to support the injured arm with the uninjured one. Place some padding between the injured arm and across the chest; a small towel will do. Then apply an arm sling (see Figure 15). To ensure the fracture is fully supported, you can apply a folded bandage across the sling and tie it around the child's arm and chest. Then take the child to hospital.

one-minute wonder

Q You mention that when treating a child with a fracture you may have to treat for shock. The treatment for shock involves raising the child's legs. How can you do this if the child has a fractured foot or leg?

A Yes, the treatment for shock does involve raising the legs. In the situation you describe, you should only raise the uninjured leg.

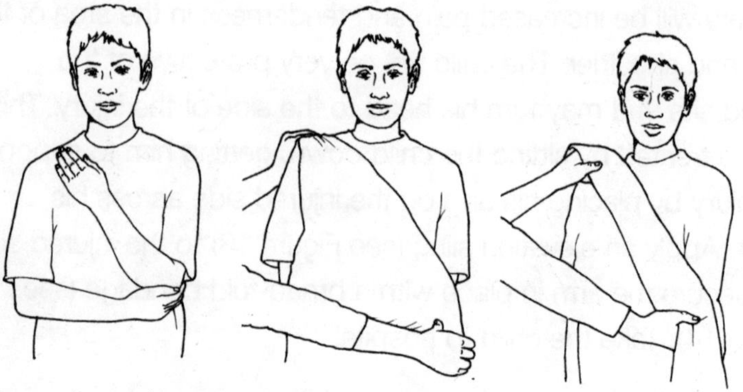

(a) Elevate and support the arm on the uninjured shoulder. Drape the long edge of the triangular bandage over the uninjured side and fold it under the injured arm.

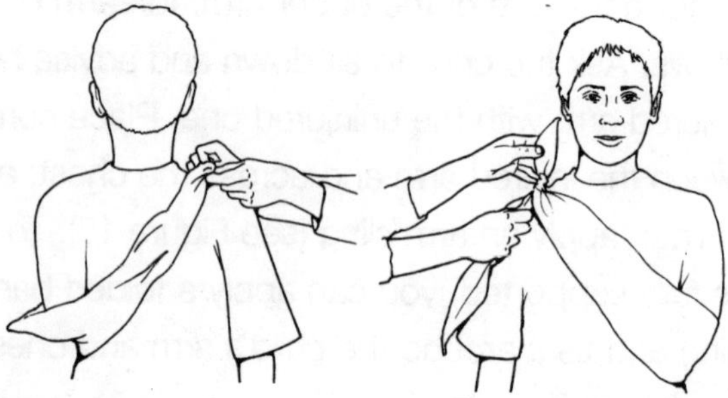

(b) Tie both ends of the bandage on the shoulder on the injured side.

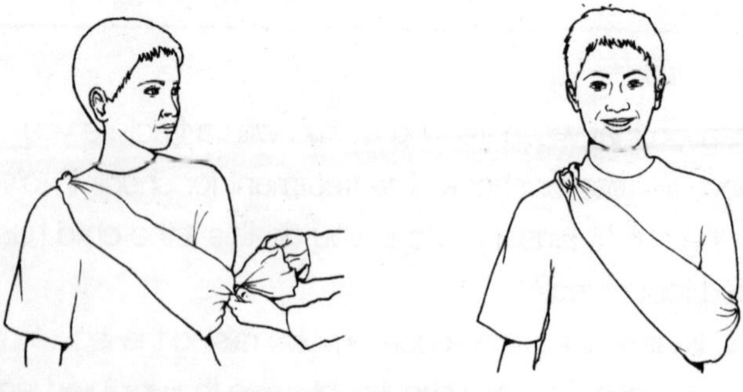

(c) Twist, tuck and pin excess fabric at the elbow.

Fig 13 An elevation sling

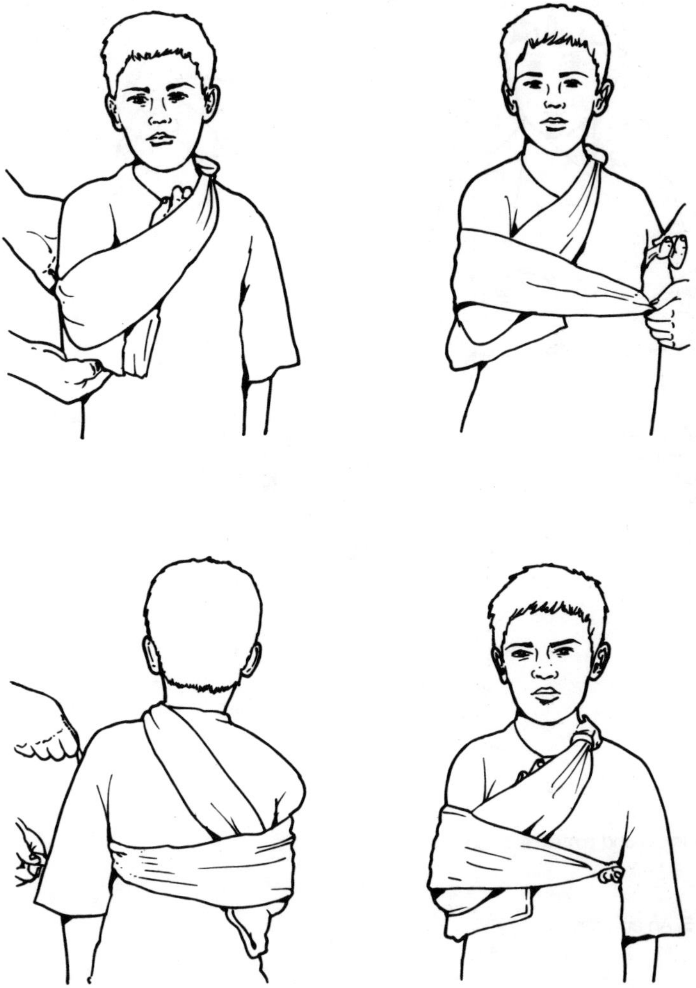

Fig 14 How to secure an elevation sling in place with a broad-fold bandage

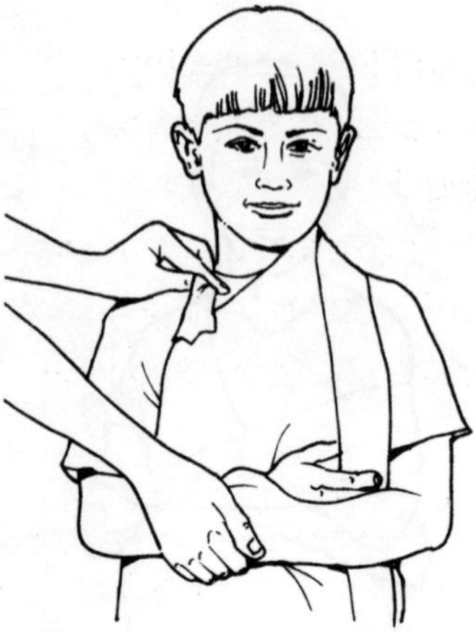

(a) Drape the triangular bandage between the arm and chest and around the neck on the injured side.

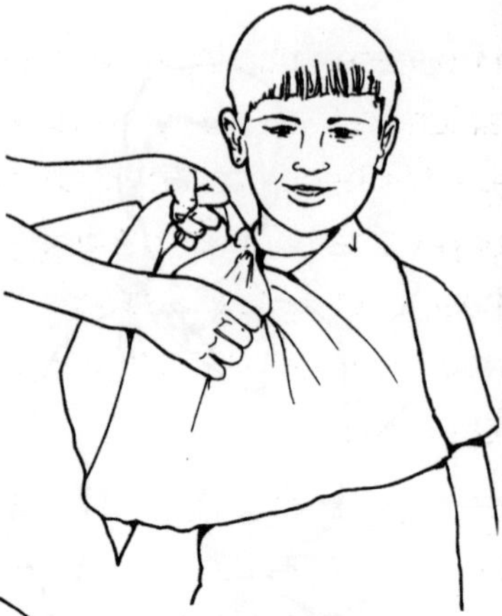

(b) Lift the bandage over the injured arm and tie both ends at the shoulder.

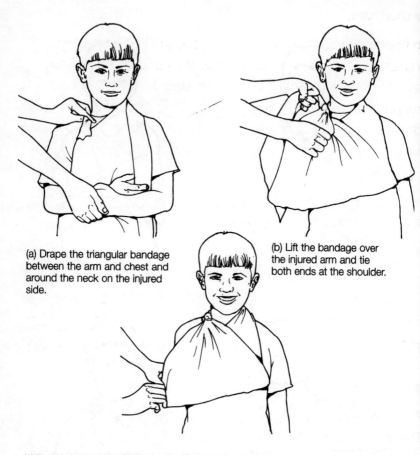

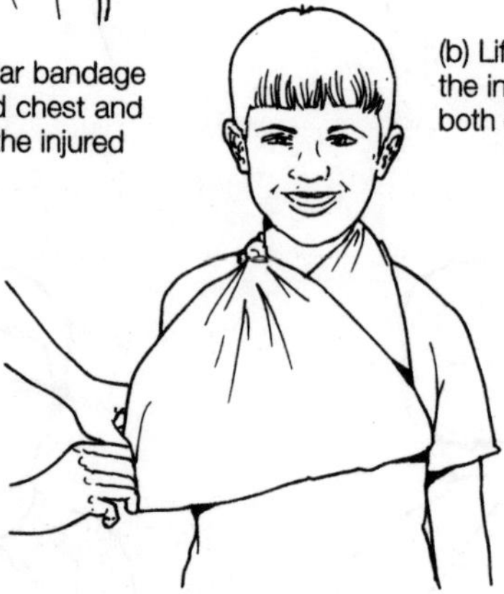

(c) Tuck in and pin excess fabric at the elbow.

Fig 15 An arm sling

broken hand

In the case of an injury to the hand, resulting in a suspected fracture in this area, you should wrap the hand in cotton wool, raise the hand and apply an elevation sling. For additional support, tie a folded bandage around the child's injured arm and chest. In the case of suspected broken or disclocated fingers, wrap the fingers in cotton wool and apply an elevation sling (see Figure 13).

---

key skills

If you suspect a closed fracture:

- try and avoid moving the person
- support the site of the injury
- arrange for the person to be moved to hospital.

---

open fractures

An open fracture can often result in significant blood loss. Therefore, your aim is to prevent the loss of blood, and to try and avoid the wound and exposed bone becoming infected. First control the bleeding (see Chapter 3), but avoid putting pressure directly on an exposed bone. If the bone is protruding above the surface of the skin, you should place rolls of clean material each side of the bone and bandage over the pads. If the site of the injury is the arm or leg, immobilize the limb as described above.

key skills

Treat any blood loss, cover the wound and bone and call for an ambulance.

dislocation

A dislocation occurs at a joint and usually results from a strong force pulling the bones apart. It most commonly involves the shoulder, fingers or toes. The history of the accident is a good indicator to whether a child has suffered a dislocation. If there is a dislocation, you may see swelling and bruising at the joint, and the child will be in intense pain. You should prevent unnecessary movement of the affected joint, and arrange for the child to be moved to hospital. Advise the child to support the injury in a position that is most comfortable for him and, if it's a shoulder injury, apply an elevation sling.

one-minute wonder

Q I was told that if you dislocated a joint you could put it back in place by pulling on the injured limb. Is this true?

A Replacing a dislocated joint is a complex medical procedure and should only be attempted by appropriately qualified medical personnel.

one-minute wonder

Q My neighbours' son regularly dislocated his shoulder playing sport, but each time it happened he claimed it 'popped' back into place. Is this possible?

A Yes, there are occasions when a joint may replace itself back into the socket. However, if this occurs we suggest seeking medical advice to ensure it is properly resited.

summary

Injuries to bones, muscles and joints are not uncommon, in fact they are a part of growing up. Many of these will be minor muscle injuries that will get better with rest and by applying ice. Others will require hospital treatment. If you suspect a fracture, treat the child as if he has one; it is better to be safe than sorry.

self-testers

1 Sprains and strains are treated using the RICE procedure. What do the letters RICE stand for?

R________

I________

C________

E________

2 **Give two reasons why it is important to ensure that a child with a fracture remains as still as possible during treatment.**

3 **What do you do if a child has a fractured leg and the bone is protruding above the level of the skin?**

4 **When you are treating a child with a fracture, give two examples when you should not consider taking him to hospital using private transport.**

---

answers

1 Rest

Ice

Compress

Elevate

2 **a** to prevent further damage to the underlying tissue and blood vessels

b to reduce pain

3 If the bone is protruding above the surface of the skin, you should place rolls of clean material each side of the bone and bandage over the pads.

4 **a** if the child displays evidence of shock

b if the fracture is open

8

ponds and poolside

Drowning occurs when a child is no longer able to breathe because water has entered his mouth and he may have inhaled a small amount of it into his lungs. It is important to remember that young children not only drown in swimming pools, in the sea and in open water, but an increasing number die as a result of drowning in a paddling pool or fish pond, both of which have become increasingly popular in domestic gardens. Furthermore, babies and children can drown in a relatively small amount of water. There have been incidents where as little as 2.5 cm of water has been sufficient to cover a child's face, resulting in drowning. Some simple precautions around the house and garden could significantly reduce the number of drowning incidents at home and outdoors. Do not leave young children unattended in the bath, and leave toilet seats down as every year there are reports of young children drowning in toilets as a result of falling in head first. In the garden, ensure that fish ponds are protected by fencing or covers, and keep swimming pools and hot tubs covered when not in use. The most obvious piece of advice is to teach your child to swim when he is young.

bath time

The majority of drowning accidents that occur in the home happen in the bathroom, and some of these happen because simple advice is not followed. It is recommended that you never leave a young child unsupervised in the bath; ideally he should be with an adult. If the phone rings or the door bell goes while you're bathing your child, ask someone else to answer it or, if you're on your own, ignore it. If you think it might be really important, take the child out of the bath but wrap him up well. Many people think that they would hear their child if they got into trouble in the bath; this is not true – children tend to drown silently. There is a wide range of bathing aids you can buy to enhance your child's enjoyment in the bathroom, but it is important to remember that these are not safety devices and should not be used as a substitute for supervision. There have been some reports of parents allowing their children to use swimming flotation devices, like inflatable rings in the bath for safety purposes. These devices were not designed for this purpose and will not ensure your child's safety.

5 ● 5

how to respond to a drowning accident

In a drowning incident, your aim as a first aider is to remove the child from the water as quickly as possible. If the drowning child is in open water such as the sea, river or lake, try and rescue him by reaching him from dry land. You may be able to use a branch or throw in a float if one is available. Your priorities are to remove the child from the water, attempt to restore adequate breathing if necessary, and to keep the child warm. Call for an ambulance.

Once you have removed the child from the water, it is important to carry him with his head lower than his chest (see Figure 16). This may result in water draining from his mouth and nose. It also reduces the risk of him inhaling further water and causing a blockage to the airway. Once on dry land or out of the bath, carry out a check of the ABC (see Chapter 1, page 9). Open the airway and check the breathing. If he is breathing, place him in the recovery position and remove the wet clothing. Then cover the child with a blanket, dry towel or any dry clothing available. If he is not breathing, start resuscitation. (See Chapter 2 for resuscitation first aid.)

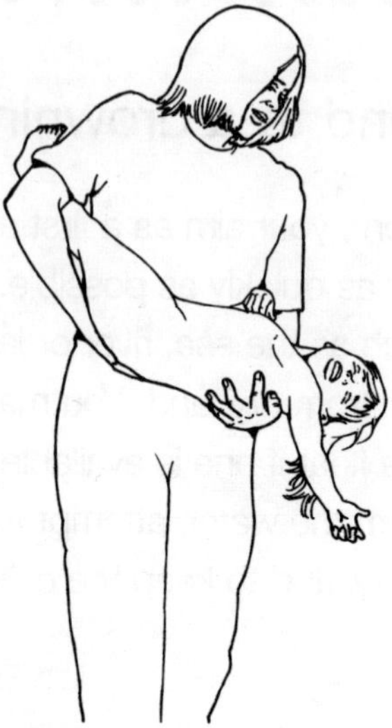

Fig 16 Carrying a drowning child

one-minute wonder

Q I was taught that you should press on a child's stomach to get the water out following a near drowning. Is this correct?

A No. Pressing on the stomach may push water into the lungs; holding the head lower than the body is the best way to allow drainage.

key skills

Remove the child from the water as quickly as possible. If clothed, remove wet clothing. If unconscious, carry out checks and be prepared to resuscitate. Call for an ambulance.

5 5

hypothermia

A prolonged time in cold water can cause death. However, this sometimes results from hypothermia rather than from drowning. We know that when a body is immersed in water it cools 30 times faster than when it is surrounded by air. Therefore, on rescuing a child from water you should observe him for signs of hypothermia. Signs include shivering, and cold and pale skin. He may appear weak, and he could possibly drift in and out of consciousness. He may also be disorientated. You should try and stop the child losing any more of his body heat, and rewarm him slowly. Replace any wet clothes with warm and dry clothing. If the child is able to walk in and out of a bath, he can be bathed in warm water, not too hot. Alternatively, put the child in a bed and give him warm drinks and chocolate. Chocolate is a high-energy food and will speed up the warming process.

key skills

To treat hypothermia, remove any wet clothing and warm the child slowly.

one-minute wonder

Q Is it OK to give a child a small amount of whisky in hot water to warm him up?

A No, the body's response to alcohol can worsen the effects of hypothermia.

one-minute wonder

Q Is it OK to use a hot-water bottle or an electric fire to warm the child?

A We do not recommend using any heat source in this situation as it may warm the child's blood too quickly.

summary

Many drowning and near-drowning incidents involving children could be prevented if young children were supervised, whether in the bath, in the pool or in the sea. We know that water holds a great appeal for children, but if your child gets into difficulty, get him out of the water as quickly as possible. Assess his ABC, and if he is breathing, keep him warm; if he is not breathing, be prepared to resuscitate.

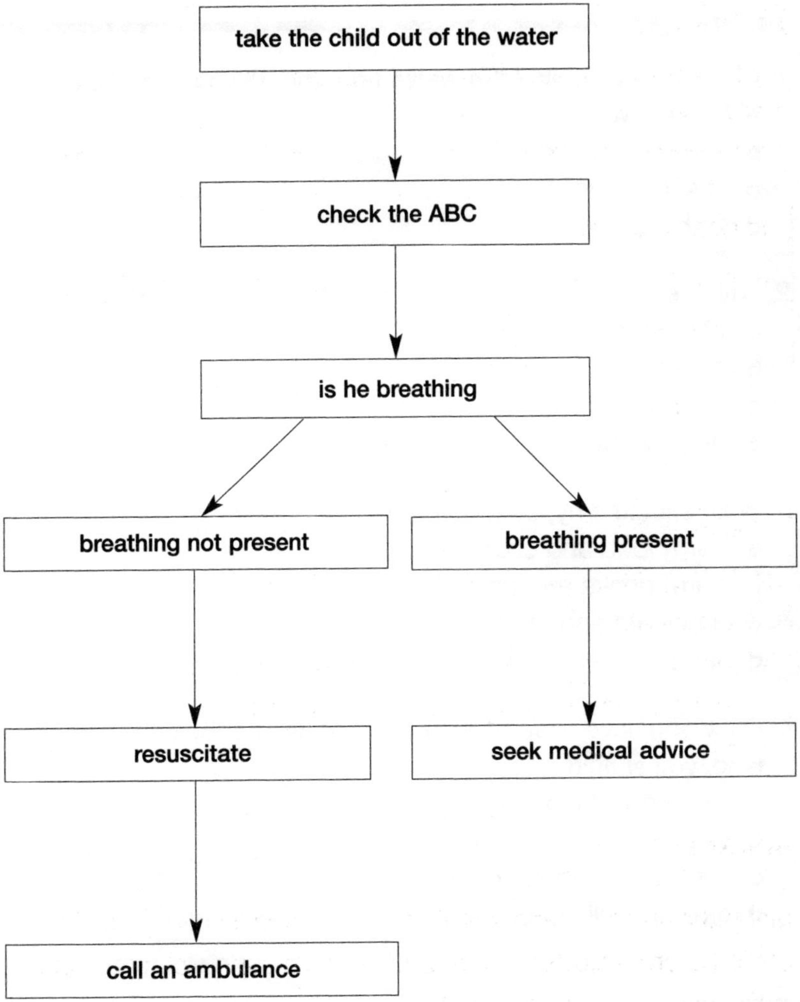

How to deal with a drowning incident

self-testers

1 **On rescuing a child from water, how should you carry him?**
- **a** head lower than chest
- **b** head higher than chest
- **c** upside down
- **d** on his back

2 **Which of the following is not a specific sign of hypothermia?**
- **a** shivering
- **b** pale skin
- **c** vomiting
- **d** weakness

3 **What should a hypothermia victim be given?**
- **a** warm food and cold drinks
- **b** warm drinks and chocolate
- **c** chocolate and alcohol
- **d** none of the above

4 **Once you have ensured your own safety and the child is on dry land, you should first:**
- **a** remove wet clothing
- **b** check ABC
- **c** assess for hypothermia
- **d** give the child chocolate

answers

1 **a**
2 **c**
3 **b**
4 **b**

9

childhood conditions

There is a large number of illnesses that your child could have in his formative years, but some of these may disappear as he approaches adult life. In this chapter we have identified some of the more common conditions, and specifically those where some basic first-aid skills could help the situation. We have tried to keep this advice simple by focusing on the care you should give while waiting for a health care professional's diagnosis and advice. Additionally, we have made reference to meningitis and febrile seizures as both of these conditions require immediate first-aid attention.

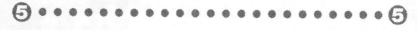

asthma

Asthma is a condition affecting the lungs and air passages that makes breathing difficult, especially breathing out. You will recognize an asthma attack because your child will have obvious difficulty breathing, and if he has a cough, you will notice him wheezing on breathing out. He will also appear anxious and distressed. If you suspect your child is having an asthma attack and has no prior history of such episodes, seek medical advice.

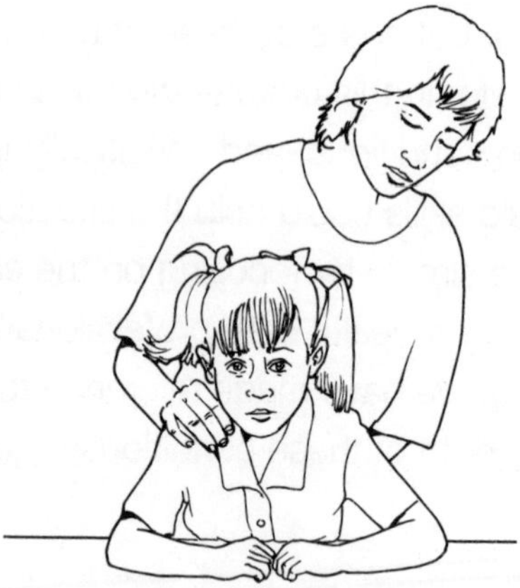

Fig 17 Sitting a child forward to ease breathing

To ease the condition, you should sit your child upright, leaning forward (see Figure 17). Make sure the room is well ventilated, and open windows and doors if necessary. If your child has had previous episodes of asthma and has medication, use it as early as possible.

key skills

To treat an asthma attack, you should:

- sit the child forward
- open the windows
- give medication.

Seek medical advice if this is the first episode or if the attack does not respond to medication.

one-minute wonder

Q Is it true that most children know how to treat themselves in the event of an asthma attack?

A Yes, assuming the children are old enough and aware that they have the condition. They usually know the precautions to take to avoid an attack, how to administer their medication, and how to position themselves to make the condition better.

It is also worth remembering two things:

1. Childhood asthma is becoming increasingly common. You may witness their first episode and have to respond. Just because they are not a known asthmatic do not regard this as an impossibility.
2. If a child has a history of a condition and he alerts you that it is a serious attack, respond to what he is telling you, call for an ambulance immediately.

epileptic seizures

Epileptic seizures fall into two main categories. First, there may be a very brief episode where the child is seen to switch off for a very short time. There may be some twitching of the face or the child may appear distracted. The child recovers very quickly. If this happens, reassure the child and arrange for him to be seen by the doctor. These seizures are often referred to as 'absence seizures', and tend to only happen to children.

Second, there are epileptic seizures. These can be recognized as the child may suddenly fall onto the floor, and sometimes he may shout or cry. As he falls, his body may become very rigid and he may arch his back and bend his knees upwards. You will notice jerking movements throughout his body; you may also observe some frothing around the mouth or the loss of a small amount of blood. The child may also lose bowel and bladder control.

The priority is to ensure the safety of the child by moving away any furniture or objects that he may injure himself on. Do not attempt to restrain the child or place anything in his mouth. Some people believe you should put a pad or a spoon in a child's mouth, but this can cause further injury or, in some cases, affect the child's ability to breath. If possible place a soft pad or flat pillow under his head for protection (see Figure 18).

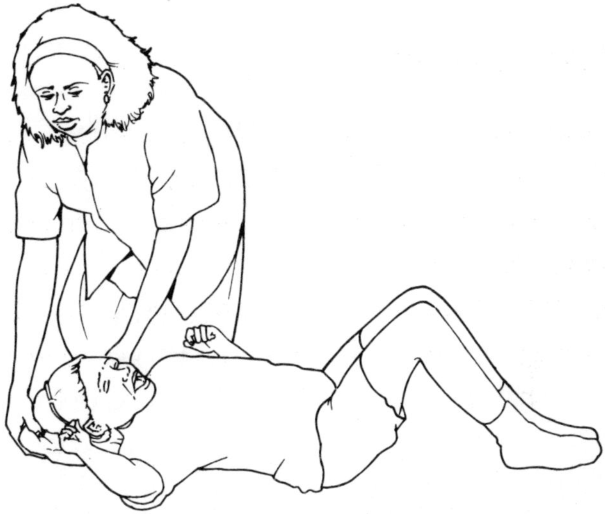

Fig 18 Protecting the head during an epileptic seizure

This phase of the seizure can last a few minutes and, once it is over, the child may appear drowsy, disorientated or unconscious. If so, check his breathing and if he is breathing place him in a recovery position (see Chapter 2, page 21). It is not uncommon for a child to sleep deeply after a seizure. You should continue to monitor his condition while he is asleep. If in doubt, seek medical advice.

If your child has a sequence of seizures, or if this is his first seizure, call an ambulance. If the child has a seizure and he is close to a wall, you should try placing some padding between the child and the wall to avoid the child injuring himself.

key skills

If you witness a child having an epileptic seizure, do what you can to ensure that he doesn't injure himself, and protect his head. If he is drowsy after the seizure, place him in the recovery position.

one-minute wonder

Q If my child has an epileptic seizure, should I place something in his mouth to stop him swallowing his tongue?

A No, the chances of a child's airway becoming blocked during a seizure are very small. There is no need to place anything in his mouth and in fact by doing so you may cause damage to his mouth, gums and teeth.

fainting

Fainting occurs when there is a temporary lack of blood supply to the brain. This results in the child becoming unconscious and falling to the ground. If your child is feeling faint, lay him down. He may have complained of feeling weak or sick, his face may be pale, and he may feel giddy.

Once the child is on the ground, raise his legs using any available object for support. To be effective, the legs must be above the level of the heart (see Figure 19). This helps because it moves the large amount of blood contained in the legs up to the brain where it is required. Loosen any tight clothing around the child's waist or neck, and ensure he has plenty of air. If he is in a room, open the windows. Ask bystanders to stand away.

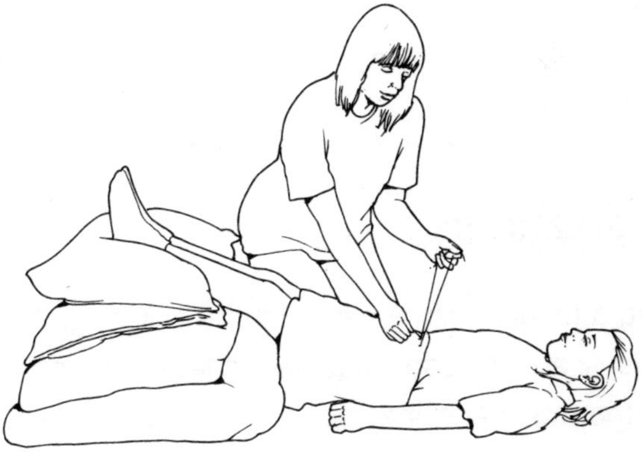

Fig 19 What to do if a child faints

The child should regain consciousness quickly. Once he does, give him a few minutes to recover before moving him. Gradually move him into an upright position by getting him to sit up first, and then stand.

one-minute wonder

Q Why does raising the legs help?

A It helps by moving the blood from the legs to the brain where it is needed.

one-minute wonder

Q I was told to sit a child up and put his head between his knees if he fainted. Is this the right thing to do?

A No. You should always lay the child down and keep his legs raised.

febrile seizures

Witnessing a febrile seizure can often be alarming. It can occur very suddenly and is associated with a fever. The child's skin will be hot to the touch and may appear red and flushed. When the seizure begins the child will involuntarily twitch his muscles, including the muscles in his face. His eyes may be fixed on the ceiling or appear up-turned. On occasions this twitching may be quite violent and the child may go unconscious. Your priority is to ensure that the child does not injure himself and to cool him so that his temperature reduces. Remove the child's clothing and bedclothes and ensure that the room is well ventilated. Using tepid water, sponge the child's body. This should reduce his temperature and the child will appear more alert. If sponging the child does not improve his condition, seek medical advice.

one-minute wonder

Q To cool my child down should I put him in a bath of cold water?

A No, you should not put the child into a bath of cold water as this can be alarming and can result in hypothermia.

meningitis

There are two types of meningitis – viral and baterial – and the signs and symtoms are similar in the early stages of the condition. The signs and symptoms of meningitis include vomiting, headache, a red or purple rash, stiffness in the neck and pain in the eyes due to light. There is a very simple test you can carry out that will help you differentiate between a rash caused by meningitis and one that appears on the skin for some other reason. This test is known as 'the glass test'. Place a tumbler type glass on the rash and apply pressure. In most cases this will cause the rash to disappear, however, in the case of meningitis it will remain.

key skills

If you suspect meningitis, do the glass test, check for the signs and symptoms described above and seek medical advice immediately.

croup

The swelling of the windpipe and voice box in children results in a condition known as 'croup'. This usually occurs at night, and the condition can be extremely alarming for a parent or carer because of the barking, whistling noise the child makes. Croup can appear to be worse if the child is crying or upset, and sometimes it is associated with the child having a cold. You will be aware if your child has croup as he will have difficulty breathing in, and he will make a short, barking cough accompanied by a croaking or whistling noise. This is a very distinctive sound and, unlike any other type of cough your child may have – some parents describe the noise as similar to the sound of a barking seal.

To treat croup, you should sit your child upright on your lap, and take him to a room with a steamy atmosphere. Keep calm and seek medical advice.

summary

Even the more common childhood illnesses can be frightening and, while many of them may require specific treatment, there are some practical things you can do to help manage these conditions. We have tried to give you some background information on these conditions and some tips on how to make the situation better. However, remember if you have any doubts about the ongoing treatment of any of these conditions, you should seek medical advice.

self-testers

1 **What are the signs of an asthma attack?**
- **a** wheezing on breathing out
- **b** wheezing on breathing in
- **c** anxiousness
- **d** coughing

2 **How should you treat an asthma attack occurring for the first time in a child?**
- **a** seek medical advice
- **b** lean the child slightly forward while he is standing in order to not obstruct the airway
- **c** sit the child down, leaning slightly forward
- **d** make sure all windows are shut to not pollute the room and cause further problems breathing

3 **What should you do when a child is having a epileptic seizure?**
- **a** try to restrain the child from falling
- **b** try to place a pillow or soft object under the head
- **c** remove any furniture
- **d** place an object in the child's mouth to stop him biting his tongue

4 **What should you do if your child feels faint?**
- **a** lie him down
- **b** raise his legs above his heart
- **c** get him to place his head between his kness
- **d** give him water to drink

answers

1 **a**, **c** and **d**

2 **a** and **c**

3 **b** and **c**

4 **a** and **b**

case studies

Jonathan's story

Jonathan was a typical six year old, slightly naughty but very likeable. He liked 'helping' his mum Kate in the kitchen to prepare food and baking. He wanted to see everything, do everything and of course taste everything. It was his insistence on seeing everything that got him into trouble. His preferred place to see his mum working in the kitchen was to sit on top of the work surface. One April afternoon, after his return from school, he sat in his usual place mixing batter for pancakes.

His mum had briefly gone into the garden to take the clothes in from the washing line. 'It must only have been a matter of seconds after I had left the room when I heard a scream that I will remember for the rest of my life,' said Kate.

On racing back into the house, Jonathan was still sitting on the work surface, but what was left of the hot water from the kettle that Kate had just made a cup of coffee with was now all over the kitchen units and the floor. Of most concern was that you could see it had spilt all over Jonathan's T-shirt and trousers. 'He was hysterical, screaming for me and holding his breath at the same time, if that's possible,' said Kate.

'I must admit I lost it a bit as well,' said Kate. 'I knew what I should do but in the panic but I didn't know what order to do it in.'

She just could not think straight. Should I take his clothes off, should I leave them on, should I take him to cold water or should I pour water over him? Should I call an ambulance or just bundle him in the car and take him to hospital? All of these questions went through Kate's mind in the few seconds after she discovered him.

She started by taking off his Jonathan's T-shirt which appeared to cause him a lot more distress. She carried him to the kitchen sink and turned on the cold tap; she then proceeded to splash the water all over him. She cannot remember how long she did it for but no more than two or three minutes. He was scalded all along the front of his stomach, down onto his thighs. The pattern of the scald was obvious from the bright marking on his skin. When Kate had finished cooling the skin, she rang her mum who lived close by and asked her to come round so that she could drive Kate and Jonathan to the hospital. Her little boy was still in pain but slightly more composed than he had been earlier.

Jonathan made a full recovery. His hospital stay lasted six weeks and the evidence of his injuries are still very obvious, but the doctors suggest they will fade with time. All the clinical wisdom is that the extent of his injuries would have been much worse if the water had been boiling and if his mum hadn't cooled his skin with cold water.

authors' observations

The way this story is told reminds us of the Morecambe and Wise sketch where Ernie claims he is a good pianist 'because I can play all the right notes, just not in the right order'. Kate did many of the right things, but not in the right order.

Once Jonathan's mum was thinking clearly, she did two of the more important things – taking off his T-shirt and cooling the area. Of course, cooling the affected area as quickly as possible is the priority. On this occasion, Jonathan was only wearing one layer of clothing and this can be removed quickly and the cooling can begin. There is no need to be concerned about the clothing being stuck to the skin – this is only a consideration with burns.

Whether you take the child to the water or the water to the child is an interesting issue. it is a decision that can only be made at the time – there is no definitive answer because the circumstances may be different. The golden rule is do whatever it takes to cool the area as quickly as possible. We note that Kate cooled the skin for two to three minutes, but all the clinical research indicates that the area should be cooled for at least ten minutes.

A large area of Jonathan's body was affected and so this was a serious injury, and therefore an ambulance could have been called and the cooling continued. Two things could have helped the pain:

1 Cling film applied to the scald will often reduce pain, prevent infection and reduce fluid loss from the body.
2 Mum could have given Jonathan some regular children's painkiller. If she had done so it is important to advise the hospital of the type, the size of dose, and the time given.

Syreena's story

Christmas 2000 was one to remember for Syreena's family. The sense of anticipation was obvious in the Joshi household, as it would be in any family home with three children under the age of six. As two-year old Syreena was the youngest, she was still easily influenced and idolized her older brother and sister. The agreement among the children was that no one would come downstairs to see what presents Santa had brought until Syreena was awake. In fact, this was not an issue on Christmas morning as the youngest member of the family was awake first and quickly went to wake her siblings.

The opening of presents resulted in the usual excitement and chaos – wrapping paper everywhere, toys all over the place, and a frantic hunt for the right size batteries. Among Syreena's presents was a tube of small plastic animals given by her aunt in Jamaica. She immediately began to play with these and ignored some of the more expensive presents.

What happened next is not clear, but Syreena's brother Guy came running upstairs shouting at his mum, 'I think Syreena's choking'. On arrival in the sitting room, Mrs Joshi's youngest was sitting on the floor.

'It was weird,' said Sandra, Syreena's mum. 'She was crying yet not making any noise, I knew something had happened but I couldn't work out what'. Sandra then noticed the small animals scattered on the floor but was becoming increasingly concerned about Syreena because she was now having difficulty breathing. Sandra looked in her mouth but couldn't see anything, and came to the conclusion that she must be choking. She put Syreena over her knees and slapped her on the back, on the third or fourth slap, 'She made a croaking noise and a little plastic dog dropped onto the floor, you cannot begin to imagine the relief' said Sandra.

When Sandra thinks back to this Christmas, she sees an image of her little girl turning blue, and giving the back slaps, each one firmer than the preceding one. 'I was becoming desperate, I was doing all this and I still was not sure if she was choking,' she said.

Syreena recovered and enjoyed the remainder of her Christmas.

authors' observations

Syreena's mum did very well. Many first-aid incidents are not witnessed by anyone and the first person on the scene has to try and work out what has happened. Looking at the scene can often give you clues. In this case there were the small animals on the floor and the distress the child was showing without making any sounds. In addition, Guy had told his mum he thought that Syreena was choking. Looking in the mouth and giving the back slaps was the correct thing to do. It is difficult to be precise about how firm the back slaps should be, but they need to be sufficiently firm to dislodge the object without injuring the child.

If you suspect that there may be some damage to the child's throat following a choking episode, it's a good idea to have him checked out by the doctor.

first-aid kit contents

There are no hard and fast rules about what should be in your personal first-aid kit. What you are most likely to need will depend on where you are and what you are doing. You may wish to keep a kit at home, another in your car, and perhaps a small version to take with you on holidays and so on. It is vital that you have the necessary supplies ready to hand for when you need them.

There are some core items that we recommend you have in any kit:

- **plasters in assorted sizes** – these are applied to small cuts and grazes. Covering the wound with a clean, dry dressing will help prevent the area from becoming infected as well as help to stop any bleeding.
- **sterile wound dressings in assorted sizes** – these are used for wounds such as cuts or burns. Place the dressing pad over the injured area, making sure that the pad is larger than the wound. Then wrap the roller bandage around the limb to secure it.
- **triangular bandages** – commonly used for slings, these are strong supportive bandages. If they are sterile then they can also be used as dressings for wounds and burns.
- **safety pins** – useful for securing crêpe bandages and triangular bandages.

- **adhesive tape** – useful to hold and secure bandages comfortably in place. Some people are allergic to the adhesive, but hypoallergenic tape is available.
- **non-alcoholic cleansing wipes** – useful for cleaning cuts and grazes. They can also be used to clean your hands if water and soap are not available.
- **roller bandages** – used to give support to injured joints, to secure dressings in place, to maintain pressure on them, and to limit swelling.
- **disposable gloves** – these single-use gloves are an important safety measure to avoid infecting wounds as well as to protect you.
- **scissors** – using a round-ended pair of scissors will not cause injury and will make short work of cutting dressings or bandages to size. It is useful to have a strong pair that will cut through clothing.
- **sterile gauze swabs** – these can be used to clean around a wound or in conjunction with other bandages and tape to help keep wounds clean and dry.
- **burn gel** – use directly on a burn to cool and relieve the pain of minor burns and to help prevent infection. Very useful if water is not available.
- **ice pack** – cooling an injury and the surrounding area can reduce swelling and pain. Always wrap an ice pack in a dry cloth and do not use it for more than ten minutes at one application.
- **tweezers** – useful for picking out splinters.

- **thermometer** – used to assess the body temperature. There are several different types including the traditional glass mercury thermometer and digital thermometer, as well as the forehead thermometer and the ear sensor. Normal body temperature is 37°C (98.6°F).
- **face shield or pocket mask** (a hygiene shield for giving rescue breaths) – these are plastic barriers with a reinforced hole to fit over the injured person's mouth. Use the shield to protect you and the injured person from infections when giving rescue breaths.
- **note pad and pen** – use the pad to record any information about the injured person that may be of use to the emergency services when they arrive. For example, the name and address of the person, how the accident occurred, and any observations. It is also useful to record vital signs so that you can monitor how well the person is doing over a period of time.
- **basic first-aid information** – a basic guide to first-aid tips, and emergency information (you can use the first aid essentials pull-out card in this book).

This is not an exhaustive list and there are many more items you may find useful to add to your kit.

Many people like to keep items such as antiseptic cream in their kits. The British Red Cross does not include anything which may no longer be sterile after the first u1se because of the risk of infection and allergies.

It is easy to make your own first-aid kit by collecting these items or, alternatively, you could simply buy a complete kit. For more information on British Red Cross kits visit **www.redcross.org.uk/firstaidproducts** or call 0845 601 7105.

The Health and Safety Executive (HSE) is responsible for the regulation of almost all risks to health and safety arising from work activity in Britain. HSE regulations concerning kit contents apply to employers. For more information about first-aid kits and training for the workplace visit **www.redcrossfirstaidtraining.co.uk** or call 0870 170 9110.

household first-aid equipment

Throughout this book we have made reference to the importance of having first-aid skills, knowledge and equipment. In terms of equipment, we recommend you have a well-stocked first-aid kit (see page 119), but we also recognize that there are emergency situations where you will not have access to any of the equipment. In such situations you will have to be creative and use whatever equipment is available to you. In this section we have identified some of the items most of us already have in our homes and suggest how they can be useful in a first-aid situation.

- **beer** – you may not always have access to cold running water when treating a burn or scald. In this case, use some other cold liquid like beer, soft drink or milk. The aim is to cool the burnt area as quickly as possible using whatever cold liquid is available. Beer can be used to cool the area while waiting for water or while walking the child to a supply of cold running water. Remember, the area should be cooled for at least ten minutes for the treatment to be effective.
- **chair** – a chair has numerous first-aid uses; when treating a nosebleed, sit the child down while pinching the nose and tilting the head forward. If you are treating a bleed from a large wound to the leg, you should lay the child down and raise the leg above the level of the heart. A chair is ideal for this purpose.

- **chocolate** – chocolate can be given to a conscious child who is diabetic and having a hypoglycaemia attack known as a "hypo". This can help raise the child's blood sugar. Chocolate can also be given to a child with hypothermia as high-energy foods will help to warm them up.
- **cling film** – cling film can be used to wrap around a burn or a scald once it has cooled. It is an ideal covering as it does not stick to the burn. It also keeps the burnt area clean and because it is transparent, you can continue to monitor the burn without removing the covering.
- **credit card** – when an insect sting is visible on the skin, a credit card can be used to scrape it away. Using the edge of the credit card, drag it across the skin. This will remove the sting. Using a credit card is preferable to using a pair of tweezers as some stings contain a sac of poison and if the sting is grasped with tweezers you may inject the sac of poison into the skin. If you do not have a credit card you can use the back of a kitchen knife or any other object similar to a credit card.
- **food bag** – a clean freezer or sandwich bag makes an ideal cover for a burn or scald to the hand. The injured part should be placed in the bag once the cooling has finished. By placing it in the bag you reduce the risk of infection and it also helps reduce the level of pain.
- **frozen peas** – frozen peas or other frozen small fruit and vegetables can be used to treat a sprain or strain. Wrap the peas in a tea towel or something similar and place them onto the injury. This will help to reduce pain and swelling. Peas are

ideal as they can be moulded around the injury more easily than bigger fruit and vegetables.

- **milk** – if an adult tooth is dislodged and cannot be placed back in its socket, it should be placed in a container of milk. This will stop it drying out and increase the possibility of it being successfully replanted by a dental surgeon.
- **paper bag** – a panic attack often results in a child hyperventilating (breathing very quickly). Reassure him and get him to breath into a paper bag, this will help to regulate and slow down the breathing.
- **steam** – if your child has an attack of croup, sit your child on your knee in the bathroom. Run the tap to create a steamy atmosphere, this may help to relieve the symptoms.
- **vinegar** – if your child is stung by a tropical jellyfish, pour vinegar over the site of the sting. This will help to stop the poison spreading around the body.
- **water** – cold running water is the preferred treatment for burns and scalds. Place the burn under a cold water tap as quickly as possible and leave it there for at least ten minutes.
- **Yellow Pages and a broom** – in the event of having to provide assistance to a child with an electrical injury, where the child is attached to the current, you can stand on a copy of the Yellow Pages to insulate yourself from an electrical shock. You should then move the electrical cable away using a dry piece of wood, a broom handle is ideal.

about the Red Cross

the British Red Cross and the International Red Cross and Red Crescent Movement

The British Red Cross is a leading UK charity with 40,000 volunteers working in almost every community. We provide a range of high-quality services in local communities across the UK every day. We respond to emergencies, train first aiders, help vulnerable people regain their independence, and assist refugees and asylum seekers.

The British Red Cross is part of the International Red Cross and Red Crescent Movement, the world's largest independent humanitarian organization. This Movement comprises three components: the International Committee of the Red Cross; the International Federation of Red Cross and Red Crescent Societies, and 181 National Red Cross and National Red Crescent Societies around the world.

As a member of the International Red Cross and Red Crescent Movement the British Red Cross is committed to, and bound by, its Fundamental Principles:

- Humanity
- Impartiality
- Neutrality
- Independence
- Voluntary service
- Unity
- Universality.

the International Committee of the Red Cross

Based in Geneva, Switzerland, the International Committee of the Red Cross (ICRC) is a private, independent humanitarian institution, whose role is defined as part of the Geneva Conventions. Serving as a neutral intermediary during international wars and civil conflicts, it provides protection and assistance for civilians, prisoners of war and the wounded, and provides a similar function during internal disturbances.

To find out more visit **www.icrc.org**

the International Federation of Red Cross and Red Crescent Societies

Also based in Geneva, the Federation is a separately constituted body that co-ordinates international relief provided by National Societies for victims of natural disasters, and for refugees and displaced persons outside conflict zones. It also assists Red Cross and Red Crescent Societies with their own development, helping them to plan and implement disaster preparedness and development projects on behalf of vulnerable people in local communities.

To find out more visit **www.ifrc.org**

National Red Cross and National Red Crescent Societies

In most countries around the world, there exists a National Red Cross or Red Crescent Society. Each Society has a responsibility to help vulnerable people within its own borders, and to work in conjunction with the Movement to protect and support those in crisis worldwide.

To find out more about the British Red Cross, visit **www.redcross.org.uk**

taking it further

useful addresses

Child Accident Prevention Trust
www.capt.org.uk
4th Floor, Cloister Court
22–26 Farringdon Lane
London
EC1R 3AJ
Tel: 020 7608 3828
Fax: 020 7608 3674
E-mail: safe@capt.org.uk

Children's health
www.netdoctor.co.uk/children/index.shtml

Government advice
www.direct.gov.uk/audiences/parents/healthandwellbeing/fs/en

Guidance on first aid for schools
www.teachernet.gov.uk/wholeschool/healthandsafety/firstaid

Meningitis Trust
www.meningitis-trust.org
Fern House
Bath Road
Stroud
Gloucestershire
GL5 3TJ
24-hour helpline:
United Kingdom 0845 6000 800;
Republic of Ireland 1800 523 196
Tel: 01453 768000
Fax: 01453 768001
E-mail: info@meningitis-trust.org

NHS Direct
www.nhsdirect.nhs.uk
Tel: 0845 4647

National Society for the Prevention of Cruelty to Children (NSPCC)
www.nspcc.org.uk/html/home/home.htm
Weston House
42 Curtain Road
London
EC2A 3NH
Tel: 020 7825 2500, Helpline: 0808 800 5000
Fax: 020 7825 2525
E-mail: help@nspcc.org.uk

International Red Cross contact details

Australia
National Office, 155 Pelham Street, 3053 Carlton VIC
Tel: switchboard (61) (3) 93451800
Fax: (61) (3) 93482513
E-mail: redcross@nat.redcross.org.au
www.redcross.org.au

Canada
170 Metcalfe Street, Suite 300 Ottawa, Ontario K2P 2P2
Tel: (1) (613) 7401900
Fax: (1) (613) 7401911
Telex: CANCROSS 05-33784
E-mail: cancross@redcross.ca
www.redcross.ca

Hong Kong
3 Harcourt Road, Wanchai, Hong Kong
Tel: (852) 28020021
E-mail: hcs@redcross.org.hk
www.redcross.org.hk

India
Red Cross, Building 1, Red Cross Road, 110001 New Delhi
Tel: (91) (112) 371 64 24
Fax: (91) (112) 371 74 54
E-mail: indcross@vsnl.com
www.indianredcross.org

Malaysia
JKR 32, Jalan Nipah, Off Jalan Ampang, 55000 Kuala Lumpur
Tel: (60) (3) 42578122/42578236/42578348/
42578159/42578227
Fax: (60) (3) 42533191
E-mail: mrcs@po.jaring.my
www.redcrescent.org.my

New Zealand
69 Molesworth Street, Thorndon, Wellington
Tel: (64) (4) 4723750
Fax: (64) (4) 4730315
E-mail: national@redcross.org.nz
www.redcross.org.nz

Singapore
Red Cross House, 15 Penang Lane, 238486 Singapore
Tel: (65) 6 3360269
Fax: (65) 6 3374360
E-mail: redcross@starhub.net.sg
www.redcross.org.sg

South Africa
1st Floor, Helen Bowden Building, Beach Road, Granger Bay,
8002 Cape Town
Tel: (27) (21) 4186640
Fax: (27) (21) 4186644
E-mail: sarcs@redcross.org.za
www.redcross.org.za

Taiwan and China
No: 8 Beixingiao Santiao, Dongcheng, East City District,
100007 Beijing
Tel: (86) (10) 8402 5890
Fax: (86) (10) 6406 0566/9928
E-mail: rcsc@chineseredcross.org.cn
www.redcross.org.cn

index